Aicha Ben Tekaya

Cardiovascular risk in patients with spondyloarthritis

Aicha Ben Tekaya

Cardiovascular risk in patients with spondyloarthritis

ScienciaScripts

Imprint

Cover image: www.ingimage.com

This book is a translation from the original published under ISBN 978-613-9-52266-8.

Publisher:
Sciencia Scripts
is a trademark of
Dodo Books Indian Ocean Ltd. and OmniScriptum S.R.L publishing group

120 High Road, East Finchley, London, N2 9ED, United Kingdom
Str. Armeneasca 28/1, office 1, Chisinau MD-2012, Republic of Moldova, Europe
Printed at: see last page
ISBN: 978-620-6-19805-5

European University Publishing

Book: Cardiovascular risk in patients with APS

ISBN : 978-613-9-52266-8

Authors: Dr Aicha Ben Tekaya

Table of contents

Chapter 1

1. Introduction :

Spondyloarthritis (SpA) is the second most common chronic inflammatory rheumatic disease after rheumatoid arthritis. This pathology has been evolving for several years, in terms of classification and nosology, as well as comorbidities, imaging and therapeutic advances. SpA encompasses different phenotypic forms (radiographic or non-radiographic axial, peripheral articular, enthesitic articular). Extra-articular manifestations (e.g. psoriasis, Crohn's disease, ulcerative colitis, anterior uveitis) help to better characterize the phenotype of the disease [1]. Although the clinical presentation varies from patient to patient, there is growing evidence of premature cardiovascular risk and increased cardiovascular morbidity and mortality in this population[2,3]. Two recent meta-analyses have suggested that increased cardiovascular morbidity and mortality in SpA is associated with early and accelerated atherosclerosis [4,5]. However, the data supporting this hypothesis come from small studies, with results that are sometimes discordant and controversial with other series that have shown no increase in atherosclerosis markers in SpA patients compared with controls [6,7].

Atherosclerosis is a chronic inflammatory disease characterized by the accumulation of plaques of lipids, calcium and cellular debris in the intima of arterial walls. This is thought to result from a complex interaction between the over-representation of traditional cardiovascular risk factors in SpA patients and the inflammatory component of the disease [1]. However, estimating cardiovascular risk secondary to atherosclerosis by calculating well-known traditional scores, such as the Framingham score, does not provide a reliable estimate of accelerated risk in these patients[8]. In this context, the development of new non-invasive imaging techniques, in particular ultrasound, has enabled a better structural and functional study of the major vascular axes, enabling precise measurements to be taken to assess sub-clinical atherosclerosis. This will enable us to improve cardiovascular risk stratification in these patients and develop preventive therapeutic strategies. The pre-atheromatous stages are: endothelial dysfunction, intimal thickening and arterial stiffness secondary to vascular injury. Current techniques for assessing sub-clinical atherosclerosis enable early lesions, such as microvascular lesions, to be detected. Ultrasound measurement of carotid intima media thickness (IMT) and detection of carotid plaques represents a non-irradiating, reproducible, rapid and reliable approach[9]. A 2ème approach is the blood flow-dependent vasodilation or FMD (Flow-Mediated Dilation) technique, which represents the most widely used method for assessing endothelial dysfunction [10]. Endothelial dysfunction is the early stage of atherosclerosis. The systolic pressure index (SPI) is a marker of cardiovascular risk and a valid method of assessing arterial stiffness [9]. The evaluation of a single parameter remains controversial.

Furthermore, to our knowledge, no study has evaluated all three of the aforementioned markers of early atherosclerosis, corresponding to different levels of cardiovascular risk: endothelial dysfunction (early-stage functional abnormality), carotid IMT (structural abnormality) and arterial stiffness in patients with SpA.

In Tunisia, no assessment of premature atherosclerosis at the endothelial dysfunction stage or of arterial stiffness has been studied in our SpA patients.

2. Pathophysiology of atherosclerosis :

Atherosclerosis is a chronic, progressive disease with a long asymptomatic phase. The mechanisms involved in inflammation appear to play a role in the atherogenesis process. The various pre-atheromatous stages are :

- **Stage 1: Endothelial dysfunction:**

The initial stage of atherogenesis corresponds to endothelial dysfunction induced by abnormal hemodynamic forces, vasoactive substances, mediators derived from blood cells or linked to classic cardiovascular risk factors[11].

The vascular wall is made up of 3 tunics, from the most superficial to the deepest: the adventitia, composed mainly of connective tissue; the media, composed mainly of smooth muscle cells; and the intima, made up of a layer of endothelial cells forming the vascular endothelium. The endothelium is a surface for exchange with blood and smooth muscle cells. Depending on the stimuli they receive, endothelial cells secrete numerous mediators, notably vasodilatory substances (NO: nitric oxide; EDHF: Endothelium-Derived Hyperpolarizing Factor; PGI2: prostacyclin) or vasoconstrictors (ET1: endothelin 1, angiotensin 2), which act on smooth muscle. Under physiological conditions, there is a balance between the production of endothelial vasoconstrictor and vasodilator factors. The endothelium thus plays a central role in the regulation of vasomotor phenomena, hemostasis, vascular permeability and the proliferation of smooth muscle cells in the arterial wall [12]. The endothelium induces arterial vasodilation through the production and release of mediators, principally NO. The latter is formed by the action of an enzyme, called NO synthase, constitutively expressed in the endothelium. NO diffuses locally, stimulating nearby smooth muscle cells. A cascade of enzymatic reactions ensues, leading to the reuptake of intracellular free calcium and the relaxation of smooth muscle cells, thus promoting arterial vasorelaxation[13]. In addition to its vasorelaxant activity, NO has many other properties, including antiaggregant and antioxidant activity, inhibition of smooth muscle cell proliferation and endothelial regeneration in response to aggression[14].

Under the influence of environmental factors, inflammation or ageing, the endothelium can be activated and undergo functional modifications that affect its various physiological functions, leading to an imbalance in the production of vasodilatory and vasoconstrictive factors, which in turn alters the vasodilatory potential of the endothelium, commonly referred to as endothelial dysfunction[11]. There is an abnormality in endothelial NO availability, and hence an alteration in endothelium-dependent vascular dilation[3]. The concept of endothelial dysfunction reflects an attenuation of the vasodilatory response to stimuli that act by releasing NO from the endothelium. **Flow-dependent vasodilation (FMD) is currently the gold standard for assessing endothelial dysfunction.** It involves the stimulation of NO production, which induces vasodilation that can be quantified[9].FMD assesses the ability of an artery to dilate after occlusion and subsequent removal of occlusion of a conductance artery. FMD measures the response of the endothelium to hypoxia artificially induced by inflating a cuff around the forearm for 5 minutes. The induced decrease in distal peripheral arterial resistance leads, after deflation of the cuff, to an increase in blood flow, resulting in NO production. The release of increased quantities of NO induces smooth muscle cell relaxation and thus an increase in vascular diameter (endothelium-dependent relaxation). Results are expressed as the difference between maximum post-occlusion diameter and baseline diameter. Endothelial dysfunction is thus the early stage of atheroma. This method reflects NO production by the endothelium, which is considered a good marker of endothelial function. Endothelial dysfunction due to lack of NO production would result in little or no arterial vasodilation. FMD is expressed as the percentage change in maximum post-occlusive diameter compared with the pre-ischemic value measured by ultrasound. The FMD threshold, below which there is a correlation with increased cardiovascular risk, is still a point of debate in the literature. Shimbo et al set the FMD threshold at 7.5% to distinguish individuals at high cardiovascular risk[15]. This threshold was soon criticized for not being predictive of future cardiovascular events. Abdessalem et al. arbitrarily set the FMD threshold for predicting myocardial infarction in Tunisian coronary patients at 10.5%[10]. Thus, the FMD threshold needs to be standardized according to the population and instrument used. In view of this discrepancy, we have considered the percentage of FMD as a continuous variable with no threshold value. FMD is strongly correlated with cardiovascular risk[10,16]. Nevertheless, FMD has shown significant intra- and inter-observer variation [17]. In our work, the assessment of intra- and inter-observer reproducibility for FMD showed a good concordance rate.

- **Stage 2: Inflammatory reaction, endothelial damage and intimal infiltration :**

Following endothelial dysfunction, an inflammatory cascade involving lipoproteins and other cells, namely macrophages, endothelial cells, smooth muscle cells and lymphocytes, will sustain the genesis of the atherosclerotic plaque according to the following sequence of events:

- LDL penetration and accumulation: LDL is involved in the first stage of the atheromatous process, accumulating in the sub-intimal layer. This is followed by oxidative modification of these LDLs by free radicals from the extracellular space, leading to secondary reactions, notably pro-inflammatory ones [18,19].

- Recruitment of macrophage monocytes and formation of foam cells: once LDL has been sequestered in the intima, circulating monocytes immobilize on the endothelial surface, pass through it, and are then activated into macrophages by contact with extracellular matrix proteins[20]. Recruitment of these circulating monocytes requires activation through the expression, on the endothelial surface, of adhesion molecules initially dependent on the presence of oxidized LDL-C in the intima, then secondarily sustained by inflammatory cytokines, expressed by plaque cells. These adhesion molecules correspond to V-CAM and I-CAM[5]. Circulating monocytes can thus adhere to the endothelial surface and enter the sub-endothelial space, where they transform into macrophages.

- Intima infiltration :

Macrophage infiltration of the arterial wall induces a chronic inflammatory response that plays a fundamental role in plaque growth. Macrophages produce numerous pro-inflammatory cytokines which increase endothelial activity, thus promoting the adhesion of new monocytes and their passage between endothelial junctions[21,22]. Lipids, initially essentially intracellular, become extracellular and aggregate to form a lipid cluster.

High-definition ultrasound of the carotid arteries enables us to identify areas of parietal thickening and non-occlusive plaques representing the early stages of atherosclerosis. In B-mode ultrasonography, the anterior and posterior walls of the common carotid artery present two echogenic lines, corresponding to the high contrast of the interfaces bounding the lumen and intima on the one hand, and the media and adventitia on the other. These lines define the IMT. This stage of intimal wall infiltration has been assessed by ultrasound measurement of the IMT. The IMT is a morphological measure providing a structural assessment of the pre-atheromatous state, while the FMD assessing the ED represents a functional abnormality. It is a reliable validated measure for predicting cardiovascular risk. A recent meta-analysis involving 119 randomized controlled trials and 100,667 patients concluded that a significant reduction in ADR progression would be proportionally correlated with a reduction in cardiovascular risk[22]. Overall results showed that each 10 µm/an reduction in ADR progression was associated with a relative reduction of around 9% in the incidence of cardiovascular disease.

- **Stage 3: Atherosclerotic plaque progression and arterial stiffness :**

A muscular fibrous cap is then formed from smooth muscle cells and extracellular matrix proteins (collagen, elastin, proteoglycans), isolating the lipid center from the arterial lumen.

An influx of pro-inflammatory cytokines such as TNF alpha, Interleukin-1 (IL- 1) etc., will induce plaque cells to produce metallo-proteinases responsible for enzymatic degradation of the extracellular matrix and consequent embrittlement of the fibrous layer. Macrophages are also responsible for plaque embrittlement via phagocytosis and the production of metallo-proteinases, leading to atherosclerotic plaque instability[23].

In the long term, calcific infiltration of the internal elastic boundary begins, progressively extending into the media and leading to calcification of the plaque, thus contributing to arterial stiffness. The method used to assess arterial stiffness was ultrasound measurement of IPS.

Asymptomatic peripheral arterial disease secondary to asymptomatic but hemodynamically significant stenoses can be detected using SPI [9]. Compared with angiography, the sensitivity of SPI was 90% and specificity 98% for stenosis of 50% or more in leg arteries[24].According to a meta-analysis that applied at least three different methods of calculating SPI, patients with SPI<0.9 or >1.3 were at high cardiovascular risk[25]. A low SPI was associated with a fourfold increased risk of cardiovascular mortality within 10 years.

❖ Morbidity-mortality and cardiovascular risk in SpA:

Atherosclerosis remains a cornerstone in the pathogenesis and prognosis of cardiovascular disease. This process appears to be accelerated in inflammatory rheumatic diseases, including SpA. SpA is associated with increased cardiovascular morbidity and mortality. Indeed, cardiovascular comorbidities have been considered the leading cause of death in SpA patients[26-29].

Literature data do not allow us to confirm this information with certainty. However, current arguments point to an increase in SVR. Some authors have shown that cardiovascular events (ischemic coronary heart disease, stroke, peripheral arterial disease) are more frequent in SpA patients than in the general population[30-32]. The risk of an acute coronary episode was considered increased even for the youngest or newly diagnosed patients[33].

However, some studies have not demonstrated a significant increase in cardiovascular morbidity in SpA compared to the general population such as that done by Brophy. s et al in 2012 finding no statistically significant increase in the rate of myocardial infarction compared to people without SpA [RD 1.28 (95% CI :0.93 to 1.74) P 0.12] [34].

Chronic inflammatory rheumatic diseases must be considered as independent cardiovascular risk factors. Combined with traditional risk factors, there are factors specific to these pathologies that explain the increased number of cardiovascular events and reduced life expectancy in these patients. Not all of these specific factors have been identified, but it is clear that systemic inflammation plays a decisive role. Under physiological conditions, hemodynamic factors (blood pressure, blood flow) are the major determinants influencing the biology of the endothelium, either directly through variations in blood flow (mechanical stimuli), or indirectly through local changes in chemical factors (chemical stimuli).

Some authors have attempted to confirm this theory by measuring certain serum markers of inflammation. Stanek et al demonstrated significantly higher levels of oxidative stress parameters and sCD40L (soluble CD40 ligand) in 48 SpA patients compared with 48 age- and sex-matched controls[19]. The ligand forming the CD40/CD40L dyad is widely expressed in cells of the vascular system and plays an important role in a variety of inflammatory reactions, so that CD40L is currently recognized as a thrombo-inflammatory molecule predictive of cardiovascular events. Indeed, CD40L concentration is increased in patients with carotid artery occlusive disease and may also be predictive of cardiovascular events[35].

3. Choice of 3 ultrasound methods :

The choice of these techniques was motivated by the following arguments:

- These are simple, cost-effective techniques that do not require a complex technical platform and can therefore be reproduced in everyday practice.
- These are non-invasive measures devoid of risks or complications requiring close patient monitoring.
- Reliability: each technique provides information on a key pathophysiological mechanism of atherosclerosis, and therefore an optimal assessment of vascular status in the population studied. EIM is a witness to sub-clinical atherosclerosis via intimal infiltration, FMD reflects endothelial function, while IPS informs us about arterial stiffness and atherosclerosis simultaneously.

The 3 ultrasound variables measured (FMD, EIM and IPS) assess the various pre-atheromatous stages, which play a key role in the detection of subclinical atherosclerosis. They are thus considered predictive markers for the occurrence of cardiovascular events. Figure 37 illustrates the progression of atheroma.

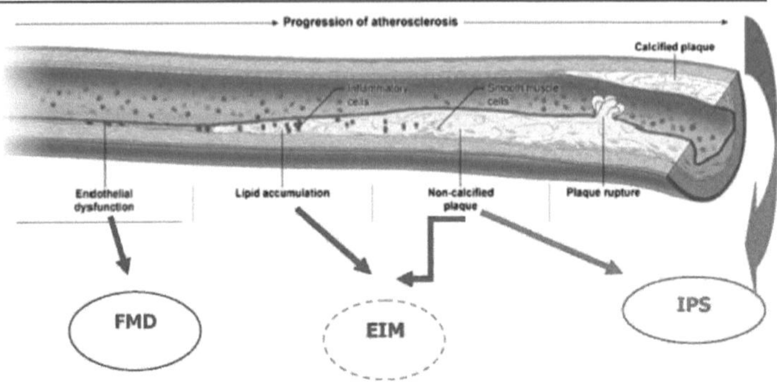

Figure: The role of ultrasound parameters in assessing the stages of the atheromatous process.

4. Ultrasound assessment of intima media thickness in SpA patients and comparison with controls :

The median mean CCA ADR was 0.55mm (IQR 25-75%; 0.48-0.62). Pathological ADR (ADR>0.7mm) was observed in 7 patients, i.e. 15% of all patients. When comparing ADR values between SpA patients versus healthy controls, right, left and mean CCA ADR values were significantly higher in SpA patients ($p<0.0001$). Thus, SpA patients had more marked subclinical atherosclerosis compared with healthy controls. We have demonstrated that our SpA patients present an increased cardiovascular risk, despite being predominantly young patients with a median age of 36 years and a predominant age class between 30 and 39 years, and having no known cardiovascular risk factors.

Our results are in line with the majority of studies that have observed a significantly greater carotid IMT in SpA patients compared with controls. Table XXXIV summarizes data from various studies, particularly those published after the latest meta-analyses, comparing carotid ADR in SpA and healthy subjects.

Two meta-analyses of the literature concluded that pathological elevation of carotid IMT was significantly higher in SpA patients than in controls, indicating that SpA is associated with sub-clinical atherosclerosis[4,5]. It is important to point out that the meta-analysis by Yuan et al, included 24 articles in which the maximum number of SpA patients recruited without cardiovascular risk factors was 67 patients (the number of subjects varied between 17 and 67 patients). This is a further argument in favour of our sample of 47 SpA patients without cardiovascular risk factors being sufficiently representative.

From another point of view, the presence of an increase in ADR does not in itself suggest that there is also an increase in atherosclerosis, but it may be associated with sub-clinical vasculitis and/or wall hypertrophy[56].Apart from any cardiovascular risk factor, inflammation in itself contributes to arterial remodelling by accelerating the various stages of atherosclerosis. However, no statistically significant difference in ADR between patients and controls was found in the studies by kaplanoglu et al , Kucukali et al, choe et al involving 38 patients/49 controls, 43 patients/41 controls and 28 patients/27 controls respectively. The small size of these series could explain these findings[7,37,38].

Factors influencing ADR :

Some authors have shown no significant difference in terms of increased carotid IMT between patients and healthy controls[7,36]. However, subgroup analysis according to SpA activity showed that ADR was significantly higher in active SpA or SpA with BASDAI>4. This fact (carotid ADR was influenced by inflammation parameters (BASDAI>4 or elevated CRP) was also observed in the results of the meta-analysis by Yuan et al, and in the series by Hatipsoylu E et al and Choe YJ et al[6,38]. ADR was not associated with CRP or disease activity scores. This is in line with the majority of findings in the literature[23].

Two Spanish studies, of which the most recent published in 2021 was multicenter and non-comparative (806 SpA) and 2ème was comparative, had revealed that 34 to 40% of axial SpA initially classified as moderate cardiovascular risk according to SCORE were reclassified as high cardiovascular risk after ultrasound evaluation measuring carotid IMT. Factors predictive of this reclassification were traditional risk factors (age, CLDL) and disease-related factors (BASFI ≥3.6; sedimentation rate ≥ 12 mm at diagnosis)[8,31].

A Giolloet al had also carried out a non-comparative longitudinal study with follow-up of carotid ADR progression over a mean duration of 13.5 ± 3.6 months in 66 SpA patients. Accelerated atherosclerosis was evidenced by carotid ADR progression of 0.01

mm/year. Predictors of this progression were impaired initial renal function and the presence of syndesmophytes[39].

Finally, our model suggests that the determinants of subclinical atherosclerosis as evidenced by carotid ADR are rather traditional cardiovascular risk factors (age, creatinine, TC). This was also suggested by the findings of Hatipsoylu et al, who considered that there was insufficient evidence to support the hypothesis of subclinical atherosclerosis influenced by high SpA activity or inflammation parameters[6]. The increased risk of atherosclerosis is most likely multifactorial in SpA patients, but the extent to which disease activity with inflammation contributes to increased atherosclerosis is controversial. Similarly, Mendonça JA et al and Perrotta FM et al had shown that ADR was also correlated with age[23,40].

J Rueda-Gotor et al were looking for an explanation for the acceleration of atherosclerosis in SpA. They assessed serum levels and the polymorphism of vaspin (a novel anti-inflammatory adipokine). No significant association was observed between ADR measurements and vaspin at either genetic or serological level[8].

The absence of atherosclerotic plaques in these patients can be explained by their relatively young age, with a median of 36 years. An interaction between age and chronic inflammation has been described[41]. Indeed, the presence of plaque is considered to be an advanced stage in the atheromatous process, compared with the elevation of ADR, due to the cumulative effect of several pro-atherogenic factors. Only one study was carried out on patients with high disease activity and an average age of over 50 years. In this study, the prevalence of carotid plaques was significantly higher than in controls[42].

5. Flow-dependent vasodilation technique :

For the second ultrasound measurement, we found a decrease in the percentage of FMD in patients compared with controls. This decrease was statistically significant, with a value of $p<0.001$. This confirms that the endothelial function of our patients is impaired compared with control subjects. These results were in line with those reported in the literature. The study of endothelial dysfunction by measuring FMD during SpA has been little studied[43- 45].however, there are 2 systematic reviews that had concluded to a significant decrease in FMD in SpA patients compared to healthy controls. The increased risk of endothelial dysfunction was directly correlated with sub-clinical atherosclerosis, and hence with a high cardiovascular risk[5,31].

Sari et al, studied FMD in 54 Turkish SpA patients compared with 31 controls free of traditional cardiovascular risk factors[46]. They found a significant drop in FMD values in patients, with a mean of 14.1% versus 17.6% in controls (p=0.03). Verma et al found a significant drop in FMD values estimated at 7.35% in 30 patients versus 10.27% in 25 controls, with a p value of 0.002[70]. Another Hungarian study showed a significant drop in FMD with a mean of 6.85 ± 2.98% in 43 SpA patients versus 8.30 ± 3.96% in 40 control subjects (p=0.005)[47].

In addition, Bodnar et al found a negative correlation between FMD and ADR[48]. We found a significant negative correlation between FMD and left ADR with medium strength, in contrast to medium ADR and right ADR. Thus, the higher the carotid ADR, the lower the FMD.

In order to determine the mechanism of endothelial dysfunction in SpA, some authors have conducted studies of vascular endothelial biomarkers. Verma et al found significantly lower serum levels of EPC (Endothelial progenitor cells), a serum marker of vascular endothelial repair, in SpA patients compared with healthy controls, indicating impaired endothelial function in SpA[50].

Another marker of endothelial function, asymmetric dimethylarginine (ADMA), an endogenous NO inhibitor, was significantly elevated in the blood of SpA patients[51,52]. This may be implicated in the mechanisms of endothelial dysfunction in SpA.

Przepiera-Bqdzak et al, found significantly lower serum levels of Endothelin-1 (ET-1) in SpA patients than in controls[54,55]. Wang et al, demonstrated that in SpA patients, serum levels of vaspin were significantly decreased and strongly associated with impaired endothelial function as measured by FMD[56].

6. Systolic pressure index :

Comparison of SPI values between SpA patients and controls revealed a trend towards higher left SPI values in patients with a median of 1.20 compared to control subjects with a median of 1.15, with a statistically significant difference (p=0.048). We found no significant difference in mean and right SPI between patients and controls.

Further analysis of the SPI distribution, focusing on the SPI>1.3 subgroup, which represents a marker of cardiovascular risk, showed that 11 patients had an SPI >1.3, compared with just one control. This increase in SPI values reflects a trend towards arterial incompressibility that is more evident in SpA patients than in the general population. An SPI >1.3 indicates arterial incompressibility or arterial stiffness by mediacalcosis mechanism, and is associated with increased cardiovascular mortality[57].

To our knowledge, this trend towards peripheral arterial incompressibility is a new finding. It has not previously been described in SpA. Published data from other inflammatory diseases such as rheumatoid arthritis and systemic lupus erythematosus indicate that arterial incompressibility results from medial arterial calcification, also known as Monckeberg sclerosis, under the influence of chronic inflammation, independently of traditional cardiovascular risk factors[57,58].

The impact of inflammation on arterial calcification is controversial. Some authors have studied the effects of cytokines on the expression and activity of alkaline phosphatase (ALP) [59,60]. Indeed, PAL is an enzyme that hydrolyzes pyrophosphate ions, potent inhibitors of mineralization, and therefore capable of inducing calcification in tissues rich in collagen fibers. Ding et al, showed that TNF- α and IL-1β stimulate PAL expression and activity independently of the osteoblast transcription factor RUNX2 [59]. This hypothesis was conceivable since TNF-α stimulates PAL expression in vascular smooth muscle cells and TNF-α blockade by infliximab specifically inhibits vascular calcification in the Ldlr/diabetes mouse model [60,61]. In this hypothesis, cytokines may stimulate ectopic calcification of collagen and this calcified matrix, in turn, may induce the calcification process, in the arterial wall. However, this hypothesis was refuted by Lencel et al, who found that TNF-α and IL-1β inhibited alkaline phosphatase activity in mouse entheses in situ, as well as in mouse and human chondrocytes, thus concluding that inflammatory cytokines had no direct effect on fibrocartilage and vascular collagen mineralization[62].

Dewi Guellec et al evaluated the value of measuring SPI in 100 RA[63]. An SPI>1.3 was noted in 5 patients, and was significantly associated with diabetes.

Taking the 2ème category of IPS<0.9, we found it to be present in 4% of SpA patients, compared with 0% of healthy controls with asymptomatic peripheral obliterative arteriopathy of the lower limbs. Thus, SpA patients with no cardiovascular risk factors are at risk of peripheral arterial disease of the lower limbs. To our knowledge, only 1 study has evaluated SPI in psoriatic arthritis[64]. In this study, Billim et al. measured SPI in 51 psoriatic arthritis patients versus 50 age- and sex-matched controls with no cardiovascular risk factors. Patients had a lower right SPI (median, 1.05 vs. 1,1, p<0.01), lower left SPI (1.04 vs. 1.09, p<0.01) and lower overall SPI (1.03 vs. 1.09, p<0.01) compared with healthy subjects. This correlated well with age and disease activity score. Del Rincon I et al found a higher prevalence of arterial incompressibility and peripheral arterial disease in RA patients compared with healthy controls[65].

From a global point of view, the measurement of SPI is another argument in favor of the increased incidence of sub-clinical atherosclerosis in patients with either arterial incompressibility or peripheral obliterative arteriopathy of the lower limbs.

7. Study of the parameters influencing the three ultrasound measurements in patients :

7.1. Patient parameters :

❖ Age :

Age was positively correlated with ADR with good linearity, and negatively correlated with FMD with poor linearity. Moreover, median carotid ADR increased significantly every 10 years. In multivariate analysis, age was the predictive factor most associated with increased carotid ADR. This finding was in agreement with the various studies that had confirmed the correlation respectively positive for ADR [66-84] and negative for FMD [37,84]. Svanteson et al, investigating factors predictive of the risk of a coronary event in 86 rheumatic patients (rheumatoid arthritis, SpA, psoriatic arthritis), concluded that age had the highest positive predictive value [86]. The predictive equation for the risk of a coronary ischemic event associated age ≥55 years, carotid IMT≥0.7 mm) and existence of atheromatous plaque with IMT≥1.5 mm (OR: 8.96, 95% CI 1.68 to 47.91), p<0.05.

However, there were discrepancies in the association between age and FMD. Bodnar et al found no correlation between FMD and age, but reported that this measure is a "snapshot" of endothelial function and does not reflect the progressive evolution of cardiovascular risk[71]. The same is true of Sari et al, who consider endothelial dysfunction to be an early stage in atherosclerosis, occurring well before structural change [69].

❖ Genre :

With regard to gender, we found no significant association with ADR and SPI. On the other hand, FMD values were significantly better in women. Celermejar et al related this difference to the pattern of changes in arterial physiology[87]. In men, the endothelial response declines progressively after the fourth decade, whereas in women, vascular physiology remains unchanged for a further 10 years. Thereafter, the decline is more rapid so that endothelial dysfunction would be similar in almost all subjects at age 65. Moreover, this gender difference could be explained by hormonal status. In VIVO, estrogen has been shown to play a protective role against atherosclerosis and vascular senescence [49,88]. After the menopause, rudimentary estrogen levels are associated with vascular decline [87].

❖ Profession:

ADR varied significantly with occupation. The most altered values were found among the unemployed. This could be explained by poor socio-economic conditions and ongoing stress. An Iranian study showed that unemployment prior to stroke was associated with an increased risk of 1- and 5-year stroke mortality[89]. The best FMD values were found in students, who are generally younger and have fewer stressful daily conditions.

❖ Marital status :

FMD was significantly associated with marital status. Married subjects showed the most altered percentages compared to single and divorced subjects who had better FMD. In contrast to our results, Manfredini et al, Celeng et al found better indices assessing subclinical atherosclerosis in married subjects [90,91]. Perhaps these results can be explained by family stress, daily demands, marital conflict and parental duties, which could lead to a poorer cardiovascular prognosis. The rheumatic patient has several constraints and a continuous stress on the one hand his rheumatism, the management of his inflammatory flare-ups including pain, insomnia, stiffness, functional impotence and on the other hand conjugal, parental and professional obligations, hence the importance of regular accompaniment and psychoeducation.

❖ Blood pressure :

Despite the non-inclusion of patients with known arterial hypertension, systolic blood pressure figures were positively correlated with ADR with good linearity and negatively correlated with FMD with poor linearity. Thus, elevated systolic blood pressure is accompanied by endothelial dysfunction. Blood pressure is a known risk factor for endothelial dysfunction and cardiovascular risk. Indeed, in the course of hypertension, a continuous rise in pressure in the microvascular system leads to premature aging and increased turnover of endothelial cells. The vascular endothelium has a reduced capacity to release EDRF (endothelium-dependent relaxing factor), resulting in impaired vasoconstriction. Hypertension has also been linked to low NO levels and increased vascular production of free radicals[92].

The positive correlation between carotid IMT and systolic blood pressure was verified in other studies during SpA[93,94].

On the other hand, arterial stiffness as assessed by the BPI in our patients was positively correlated with diastolic blood pressure in a significantly moderate and weakly linear fashion. A recent Taiwanese study attempted to measure the Ankle Arm Pressure Index using systolic, diastolic and mean 4-limb blood pressure and predict long-term mortality risk. They found that diastolic pressure index <0.78 had the most sensitive predictive value for cardiovascular mortality [95].

7.2. Disease-related parameters :

❖ Age of onset of SpA and length of disease :

ADR was positively correlated with duration of disease progression, suggesting that this parameter was associated with an increased risk of developing atherosclerosis in SpA. Other authors have also reported this association[6,68,70,71,96]. Gonzalez et al found that the duration of SpA was associated with the development of atherosclerotic plaques [68]. However, Peters et al, showed that the age of the disease had no influence on ADR[51]. This controversy between studies may be explained by the variability of sociodemographic parameters and heterogeneity in the distribution of patients' duration of disease progression between studies.

In addition, ADR was associated with age of disease onset. Kimhi et al found a significant association with age of disease onset in patients with psoriatic arthritis[97].

Thus, duration of disease progression and age of early onset could be superimposed, non-confounding variables.

❖ Phenotypic form of spondyloarthritis :

-There was a significant difference between the types of peripheral SpA in terms of

SPI, with a trend towards arterial incompressibility in the peripheral articular and enthesitic forms. The median mean SPI was 1.3 in the peripheral forms, suggesting that they are more associated with increased cardiovascular risk. This may be related to the reduced mobility of the lower limbs secondary to inflammatory involvement, resulting in more severe structural remodelling and, consequently, a higher incidence of mediacalcosis.

❖ Metrology of the spine :

An analytical study of the 3 ultrasound measurements showed a significant positive correlation between tragus-right and left acromion and chin-left acromion distances with IPS. Thus, cervical limitation in rotational and lateral movements is associated with increased arterial stiffness. Bodnar et al also found a positive association between cervical stiffness and arterial stiffness[71]. This team studied the association of spinal metrology with carotid IMT, FMD and VOP. The latter parameter would enable arterial stiffness to be assessed by measuring the speed at which the pulse wave propagates along the arterial tree. They demonstrated a significant positive correlation between VOP and occiput wall distance, but also with carotid IMT. Similarly, they found a negative association with Schober index and thoracic ampliation, suggesting that stiffness of the dorsal and lumbar spine was associated with an acceleration of sub-clinical atherosclerosis. These findings were not found in our patients. This discrepancy could be explained by the more altered cervical, thoracic and lumbar involvement in patients included in this study compared with our own (occiput wall distance: 8.2±8.5 cm VS 3[2-5]; thoracic ampliation 2.3±1.2 VS 4[2-6]; Shober index 2.2±1.7 VS 3[2-5]).

In addition, the mean age of patients and the duration of disease progression were more important. Also, in our series, the BASMI score was not associated with the 3 ultrasound measurements. In line with our findings, there was no significant association between FMD and spinal metrological data.

Thus, endothelial dysfunction, the early phase of atherosclerosis, was not associated with spinal limitation. Arterial stiffness, the late phase of the atheromatous process, was significantly influenced by cervical, dorsal and lumbar stiffness. Further studies are needed to better understand the underlying mechanism.

❖ Structural damage :

Structural damage was significantly associated with cardiovascular risk in our patients.

Indeed, we showed that CCA ADR was significantly associated with the presence of erosive Romanus spondylitis and ankylosis of the posterior inter-apophyseal joints. On the other hand, FMD was significantly low in the presence of vertebral squaring and syndesmophytic intervertebral bone bridges. Furthermore, FMD was negatively correlated with the mSASSS score.

The relationship between spinal structural damage and atherosclerosis has been little studied in the literature. Two recent studies concurred with our findings[60,65]. ML Ladehesa-Pineda et al, demonstrated a significant increase in atheromatous plaques in SpA compared with healthy controls, which were associated with a high mSASSS score (total, cervical and lumbar), and the existence of syndesmophytes and bone bridges[60].A Giolloet al had also conducted a non-comparative longitudinal study with follow-up of carotid ADR progression over a mean duration of 13.5 ± 3.6 months in 66 SpA. Accelerated atherosclerosis was evidenced by carotid ADR progression of 0.01 mm/year. The presence of syndesmophytes was identified as a predictive factor for this progression[65]. However, Gonzalez-Juanatey et al found no significant association between syndesmophytosis and carotid ADR[68]. There was no significant association of ultrasound parameters with the total BASRI score. This score appears to be less sensitive to radiological progression than the mSASS score[98]. Kang KY et al had shown that the number of syndesmophytes was independently associated with coronary risk in the next 10 years by the Framingham score in a cohort of 185 SpA with no known cardiovascular pathology[99]. Radiographic structural damage was significantly associated with increased cardiovascular risk: high levels of the score assessing the risk of cardiovascular death at 10 years were independently associated with the mSASSS score after mutlivariate analysis[60].

The mechanism of impact of structural damage on the progression of carotid ADR and endothelial dysfunction is still poorly elucidated. We know that in the relationship between structural damage during SpA and cardiovascular risk, there are four main confounding factors: age, smoking, CRP, NSAID use and disease duration[60]. However, ML Ladehesa- Pineda et al, demonstrated that this association was positive independently of these factors.

The following table summarizes data from various studies of associations between radiographic parameters assessing structural damage in SpA and ultrasound parameters.

Table: Association between structural damage in SpA and ultrasound parameters in the literature.

Article	Radiographic parameters	Ultrasound parameter studied	p
ML Ladehesa-Pineda 2020[60]	-mSASS. -Syndesmophytes. -Bone bridge.	**EIM**	**P<0,0001.** **P<0,001.** **P<0,0001.**
A Giollo2017[65]	Syndesmophytes	**EIM**	**P= 0,01.**
Gonzalez-Juanatey[68]	Syndesmophytes	**EIM**	NS
	-Romanus erosive spondylitis. -Ankylosis of the AP.	**EIM**	**P= 0,05.** **P=0,35.**

AP: Articular posterior; EIM: Epaisseur Intila media; FMD: Flow mediated dilation; mSASSS: modified Stoke Ankylosing Spondylitis Spine Score; NS: Not significant;

P: Degree of significance ;

❖ Hip damage:

Coxitis was frequent in our sample (53%), exceeding the average prevalence in the literature, which ranges from 19% to 36%[100].in fact, under our conditions, the Maghrebian SpA form is the most prevalent and is characterized by the frequency of coxitis[101]. The severity of disability according to Lequesne's algo-functional index was judged to be mostly moderate to severe, and the presence of coxitis had no significant impact on the 3 ultrasound measurements. Median carotid IMT was higher in cases of densifying coxitis, with a statistically significant difference on the right (p=0.02) and no significant difference on the left (p=0.166). Median FMD was lower in coxitis, with no significant difference. Median FMD was lowest (2%) in densifying coxitis on both sides, with no significant difference, suggesting that coxitis may accelerate endothelial dysfunction and subclinical atherosclerosis, particularly in densifying coxitis, the most common form. On the other hand, the left Lequesne index was significantly and negatively associated with FMD with high linearity. The results showed that the left Lequesne index was the strongest predictive factor that contributed most to the decrease in FMD.The Lequesne index was inversely correlated with FMD. Hamdi et al, showed no significant correlation between coxitis and carotid IMT in 60 Tunisian SpA patients (50% of SpAs had coxitis)[64].

To our knowledge, this was the first study to show an association between coxitis and its functional repercussions and markers of subclinical atherosclerosis. Mendonça et al performed ultrasonographic evaluation of the resistance index of the sacral and internal iliac arteries in 22 SpA patients[23]. They demonstrated a decrease in resistance that correlated with serum markers of inflammation. This decrease in resistance led to micro and macro vascular changes, thereby influencing endothelial function. Femoral epiphyseal vascularization comes mainly from collaterals of the femoral artery and secondarily from collaterals of the internal iliac artery. This hypothesis suggests that inflammatory damage during coxitis is responsible for a drop in resistance in the femoral and internal iliac arteries, leading to endothelial dysfunction. These hypotheses require further study in large North African series to determine the pathophysiological mechanism of this association.

- **Disease activity :**

The ultrasound parameters undertaken in our patients were not associated with CRP or disease activity scores. This is in agreement with the majority of results in the literature (Table XXXIV). However, subgroup analysis according to SpA activity in the series by kaplanoglu et al had shown that carotid ADR was significantly higher in active SpA or with BASDAI>4 [7]. This was also observed in the results of the meta-analysis by Yuan et al, and in the series by Hatipsoylu E et al and Choe YJ et al [4,6,58].

7.3. Biological data :

-Renal function: Creatinine correlated significantly positively with mean ADR (p= 0.009) and negatively with FMD (p =0.001). The

Multiple linear regression showed that creatinine was a strong predictor of ADR: each 1 unit increase in creatinine increased ADR by 0.002mm. Among all the extra-articular manifestations investigated, there was only a significant association between mean ADR and renal involvement. Thus, the presence of renal involvement or elevated creatinine levels was associated with increased carotid ADR and endothelial dysfunction, and thus with subclinical atherosclerosis. These findings have been reported in other studies[102,103].Giollo A et al showed that carotid ADR progression of 0.1mm/year was associated with elevated creatinine and normal initial glomerular filtration rate[65].

In fact, endothelial dysfunction as a precursor to atherosclerosis is perpetuated by numerous factors including the renal system: stimulation of the renin angiotensin system, fluid retention with glomerular sclerosis, oxidative stress, disturbances in phospho-calcium metabolism, endocrine disorders and uremic toxins[102,104,105].This fact reminds us that kidney damage represents not only a turning point in the progression of the disease, but also an additional factor that considerably increases cardiovascular risk, and necessitates the implementation of cardiovascular disease prevention measures.

-Platelets: Biologically, platelets have been significantly correlated with FMD, probably through their incorporation into inflammation and hence atherosclerosis. Moreover, endothelial cells generate endothelial progenitor cells (EPCs), which play a key role in platelet aggregation and thrombus formation[106]. This was not confirmed by Ruane-O'Hora et al, who showed that platelets did not modify FMD in Vivo [107].

-Blood glucose: Blood glucose was also significantly positively correlated with ADR and negatively correlated with FMD. Multiple linear regression showed that blood glucose was a strong predictor of FMD, with each 1 unit increase in blood glucose lowering FMD by 4.746%. Hyperglycemia and diabetes are the first known cardiovascular risk factors. We underline the importance of this result: this highly significant correlation with 2 markers of sub-clinical atherosclerosis was found in young subjects aged under 50, non-diabetic and with normal fasting blood glucose levels except for 1 patient at the upper limit of 5.91 mmol/l.

An Indian study also found a significant correlation between blood glucose and HbA1c with FMD and ADR[108]. Thus, blood glucose monitoring is of paramount importance as it correlates with ultrasound measurements in these patients who are free of FRCV.

-Lipid profile: the 2 parameters significantly and positively correlated with carotid IMT were TC and TC/HDL ratio. Multiple linear regression showed that TC was a strong predictor of ADR: each 1 unit increase in TC increased ADR by 0.034mm. The significance of these findings derives from the absence of known dyslipidemia in these patients, and the fact that only 2 of the 47 patients included had a hypercholesterolemia. These results were similar to a Chilean study which found a significant correlation of carotid ADR with TC, and the TC/HDL ratio was the predictive factor most associated with ADR[109]. We found no significant association between carotid ADR and other lipid parameters such as TG, HDL-C, LDL-C and LDL-C/HDL ratio. Results on the association between lipid profile and markers of subclinical atherosclerosis in SpA patients with no dyslipidemia differ. A comparative Spanish study showed that SpA patients had significantly more carotid atheromatous plaques and a higher carotid IMT than controls, and that 34% of axial SpA patients moved from the moderate cardiovascular risk category to the high cardiovascular risk category after this ultrasound evaluation. The factors determining this reclassification were age and LDL-C[61]. Also, Kahndelwel et al showed that there was a significant association between ADR and LDL-C [103].Skare et al[96] , Hatipsoylu et al[6] had also found a significant association between carotid ADR and triglycerides. Cure E et al concluded that there was a positive correlation between ADR and TG/HDL and TC/HDL ratios,[4] as in our series.

Several studies have found no correlation between lipid parameters and ultrasound measurements[69,70,94].

On the other hand, Kahndelwel et al also found a significant association between FMD and LDL-C[103]. Indeed, endothelial dysfunction has been correlated with cholesterol levels even when the concentration is within the normal range[110].

-CRP: These authors [57,68,93] explained the absence of a positive correlation with relatively low CRP levels [68,93]. The median CRP in our patients was 6.45. However, the meta-analysis by Yuan et al concluded that inflammation parameters (CRP) were associated with a significant increase in ADR in SpA compared with controls[4] . Similarly, Verma et al and Fischhilsher et al found a significant correlation between CRP and FMD. The role of serum markers of inflammation in the pathophysiology of atherosclerosis remains controversial [70,111].

7.4. Therapeutic data :

-NSAIDs: We found no significant association between the types of NSAID molecules and the NSAID ASAS score with the various ultrasound parameters. This was in agreement with the results of Bodnar et al in SpA[71] and Kimhi et al in psoriatic arthritis[97]. However, certain NSAID molecules have been associated with an overestimation of cardiovascular risk, such as Anti COX2 and Diclofenac[112]. Diclofenac was the most commonly used molecule among our patients (46.5%), followed by anti Cox2. Indeed, NSAIDs are a cornerstone in the treatment of SpA, especially in its axial form, which was the most frequent. The effect of NSAIDs on cardiovascular risk remains controversial. Some consider that they have a beneficial effect by reducing biological inflammation, which improves mobility and may therefore explain the reduced cardiovascular risk[50]. Others see a deleterious effect, due to the increase in blood pressure they generate. Pharmacologically, this is explained by the inhibition of cyclooxygenase 2, affecting the synthesis of prostacyclin and prostaglandin, which act as endogenous mediators of platelet activation, hypertension and atherogenesis[113].

-Anti-TNF:. The median duration of anti-TNF treatment was 36 months. For ADR, the two categories of patients had an almost similar median. The FMD of patients on biotherapy was more impaired, with a median of 12.5% compared with 15.5% of other patients, although this was not statistically significant.The median SPI of patients on anti-TNF therapy was 1.21, with a P75 verging on the upper limit at 1.33, compared with a median of 1.17 and a P75 in the normal range at 1.28. This may suggest an unchanged trend in ADR. This could suggest an unchanged trend towards arterial incompressibility despite anti-TNF therapy. However, the sample was too small and heterogeneous (18 anti-TNF+/29 anti-TNF-). The protective role of anti-TNF-alpha against cardiovascular risk via its anti-inflammatory effect is still controversial.

The absence of a significant vascular effect of anti-TNF agents on the improvement of carotid IMT has been observed in several series[6,56,114]. A randomized, double-blind Chinese study enrolled 41 SpA patients (20 anti- TNF+=Golimumab/21anti-TNF-) with 12-month follow-up via ultrasound parameters including ADR. There was a significant progression in mean ADR in the golimumab group, although maximal ADR was unchanged[115]. Another longitudinal study by Van Sijl et al[116] assessed ADR progression in 67 SpA patients treated for around 5 years with anti TNF. They found almost unchanged values in patients with good compliance, whereas the mean ADR was altered in patients taking treatment discontinuously.

On the other hand, some studies, including the meta-analysis by Yuan et al, have shown a positive effect of anti TNFs on the reduction of carotid IMT in SpA patients treated with anti TNFs compared with controls or naive anti TNF patients[4,117,118]. The mechanism of this positive effect has not been clearly elucidated. A recently published study reported a rapid and sustained reduction in complement activation in SpA patients on anti TNF, and suggested that the observed reduction in cardiovascular morbidity is partly due to its beneficial effect on complement[118]. However, the duration of anti TNF use was not reported in the study.

In contrast to our results, Vegh et al. found significant improvement in endothelial function and vascular stiffness after 12 months of Etanercept treatment in 17 of the 53 SpA patients included[114]. However, the mean ADR remained unchanged after one year.

Concerning arterial stiffness, some studies such as Capkin et al[119] , Mathieu et al[120] used pulse wave velocity. They found no improvement in PWV values at 6 and 12 months of anti-TNF treatment, despite a clear improvement in disease activity and inflammatory parameters.

With regard to the contribution of anti TNF agents to endothelial function, Szekanecz et al [121] observed a brief, transient improvement in endothelial dysfunction in patients treated with infliximab or rituximab, followed by a rapid deterioration in FMD values and a return to baseline values in the long term. The study by Gonzalez-Juanetey et al[122] of 7 RA patients concurs with his findings, explaining that the effects of infliximab on FMD were associated with inhibition of acute-phase reactant production, suppression of endothelial cell adhesion molecule production and increased serum adiponectin levels[123]. However, to the best of our knowledge, none of the studies found any alteration in FMD after initiation of anti-TNF alpha. This was re-discussed by a systematic review of the literature which identified 60 studies that examined the effects of anti-TNF agents on the sub-clinical progression of arteriosclerosis and atherosclerosis in a range of chronic inflammatory diseases. The conclusions of this review were the short-term improvement of FMD in response to anti-TNF. Results were mixed for VOP assessing arterial stiffness and largely negative for ADR. However, the quality of the studies is questionable, as they involved relatively small sample sizes and short follow-up periods[124]. Some authors have suggested that regular, concomitant consumption of NSAIDs may contribute to the increased cardiovascular risk through its prothrombotic and fluid retention effects, thus counterbalancing the effect of anti-TNF agents[93,125,126].

On closer examination of our population, the median age and duration of disease progression in the two categories (anti -TNF+/anti-TNF-) were significantly different. In anti-TNF patients, the median age was 43 years, with a duration of disease progression of 12 years. For anti-TNF-naive patients, the median age was 32 years and the duration of disease progression 7 years, with p values of <0.009 and <0.004 respectively. This must be taken into account before studying the difference.

Lipid profile and ultrasound parameters varied significantly with age and duration of disease[50]. Indeed, despite the longer duration of disease and greater median age of patients on anti TNF-α, lipid profile and disease activity scores were comparable between the 2 subgroups. We found no significant difference between anti-TNF and non-anti-TNF patients in terms of all lipid parameters (TC, TG, LDL-C, HDL-C, TC/HDL-C ratio and LDL-C/HDL-C ratio), and in terms of ultrasound measurements. This suggests long-term stability of the lipid profile.

Based on these two studies and our own, we cannot conclude that anti-TNFs have a positive vascular effect, but rather that they slow the progression of markers of sub-clinical atherosclerosis. In addition, some authors argue that anti-TNFs probably have an inhibitory effect on endothelial dysfunction, given that this is the first stage of atherosclerosis, hence the importance of detecting subclinical atherosclerosis at an early, reversible stage.

Like our sample size, the number of series is relatively small, due to the difficulty of recruiting SpA patients free of any cardiovascular risk factors.

Chapter 2

8. Predictive factors-Multivariate analysis :

Factors predictive of increased carotid IMT were age, TC and TC/HDL ratio. For FMD, factors predictive of endothelial dysfunction were creatinine, glycemia and Lequesne's algofunctional index.

Thus, we note that models predicting sub-clinical atherosclerosis parameters are not related to disease, nor to SpA activity, but rather are traditional cardiovascular risk factors (ADR++). Moreover, this is in line with the literature as discussed above. This underlines the importance of comprehensive patient management. It is not enough to stabilize osteoarticular damage with conventional treatments or biologics. Non-active SpA may present an increased cardiovascular risk in the presence of disrupted and unaddressed traditional cardiovascular risk factors. Regular cardiovascular assessment is essential.

The link between the functional impact of coxitis and endothelial dysfunction, the first stage in atherosclerosis. Coxitis is often early onset and very frequent in our patients. Its management is quite delicate, and the decision whether to start or switch to another biotherapy or indicate surgical treatment often requires a multidisciplinary meeting. Now, if we know that active coxitis could worsen endothelial dysfunction and contribute to the progression of sub-clinical atherosclerosis, its management becomes urgent and should be considered independently of scores for disease activity or remission of other axial or peripheral involvement.

9. Recommendations-Prospects

It has been shown that SpA patients who are young (<50 years) and have no known cardiovascular risk factors, and most of whom have low disease activity, have a higher risk of sub-clinical atherosclerosis than the general population. Ultrasound measurements of FMD, carotid IMT and IPS are markers of cardiovascular risk with good reproducibility, and can be used to monitor sub-clinical CV risk [31] .

Current priorities for the Tunisian rheumatologist include identifying patients most at risk of cardiovascular disease and developing preventive therapeutic strategies.

To this end, a multicenter study is needed to stratify cardiovascular risk in Tunisian spondyloarthritic patients.

We propose the following recommendations:

- Identify the patient profile: a patient with SpA is at high cardiovascular risk if he or she presents at least :
  - Advanced age of onset of SpA
  - A traditional cardiovascular risk factor: disturbance of glycemia, lipid balance, high blood pressure...
  - Creatinine above the upper limit of normal
  - Spinal structural damage.
  - Coxitis.
- Establish with vascular physicians (cardiologist, angiologist, vascular surgeon) a rhythm adapted to the Tunisian patient profile for cardiovascular risk screening in terms of :
  - Traditional cardiovascular risk factors: blood pressure, glycemia, lipid profile, creatinine.
  - Ultrasound measurements: FMD appears to be the earliest parameter

  It is important to point out that EULAR has recommended an annual blood pressure test, a blood glucose test every 3 years and an LDL-C test every 5 years, and an ultrasound scan of the supra-aortic trunks every 5 years. This does not seem appropriate for the Tunisian SpA patient and may be insufficient[127].
- As part of the overall management of SpA patients, it would be ideal to propose an annual assessment during a therapeutic education session:
  - Diet assessment
  - Offer antioxidants as a simple preventive measure:
    vitamin E, vitamin C, turmeric... Indeed, NO inactivation due to increased free radical production in the vessel wall is an important mechanism of endothelial dysfunction[92]. Consequently, great interest has been shown in antioxidants, such as vitamin E and vitamin C, as they can scavenge oxygen free radicals, and thus improve endothelial function. A single oral dose of vitamin C (2 g) improved FMD in patients

describing a

inflammation[128]. A curcumin-based diet appears to have an anti-oxidant and anti-inflammatory role, helping to optimize endothelial function. A meta-analysis of 5 randomized clinical trials demonstrated a significant effect of curcumin-based preparations in improving FMD compared with placebo, and hence endothelial function[129].

■ Draw up a physical activity schedule and submit it regularly to your rheumatologist and physiotherapist.

■ Strict control of modifiable cardiovascular risk factors. In collaboration with vascular physicians, establish an algorithm for statin prescription thresholds. It is now well established that this treatment reduces cardiovascular morbidity and mortality in both primary and secondary prevention [130]. The beneficial effect of statins in primary and secondary prevention stems not only from their cholesterol-lowering effect, but also from the significant improvement in ADR progression [131], the anti-inflammatory effect by reducing CRP synthesis [132], the antiatherogenic and antithrombotic effect [133] and the antioxidant effect by reducing free radicals and thus improving endothelial function. The Tunisian rheumatologist must therefore adopt a therapeutic approach to avoid delaying the beneficial prescription of statins. A summary diagram illustrates the recommendations in figure 38.

Figure 1 : Summary of perspective recommendations for SpA patients at high CV risk.

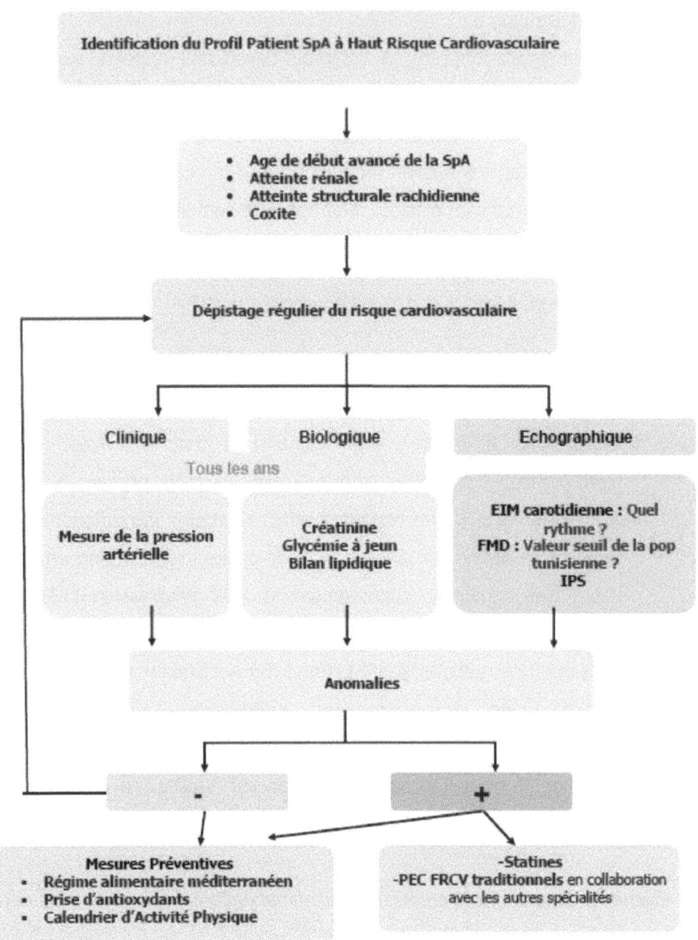

+: Presence of anomalies; -: Absence of anomalies; IMT: Intima Media Thickness; FMD: Flow mediated dilation; SPI: Systolic Pressure Index; Pop: Population; SpA: Spondyloarthritis.

10. Characteristics of epicardial adipose tissue and its role in coronary atherogenesis :

❖ Anatomical characteristics of the TAE :

WT is visceral adipose tissue located between the inner lining of the pericardium and the myocardium, in direct contact with the myocardium and coronary arteries it surrounds. It is preferentially located on the atrioventricular and interventricular sulci, on the free edge of the right ventricle and around the main coronary vessels. This means that the main coronary arteries running along the surface of the myocardium are in direct contact with the TAE.

❖ WT functional features

WT is a brown-type adipose tissue (thermogenesis), a true source of the fatty acids needed to meet the energy requirements of cardiac muscle, particularly in ischemic conditions (due to its high content of saturated fatty acids and its ability to release free fatty acids)(23).

Under physiological conditions, WT also plays a vital role in maintaining fatty acid homeostasis in the coronary microcirculation, and has thermogenic properties, protecting the myocardium and coronary circulating blood against hypothermia.

The WT is also an endocrine organ, secreting cytokines and adipokines that can diffuse freely into contact tissues such as the myocardium(24). The many hormones it produces, foremost among them the insulin-sensitizing adiponectin and leptin, have a strong influence on the body's metabolic homeostasis, acting either paracrine after diffusion into the lumen of the coronary arteries, or paracrine when secreted directly into the vasa vasorum (25).

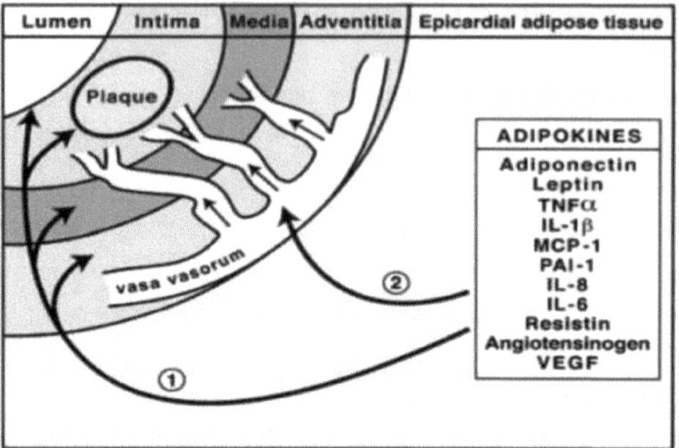

1: Paracrine signaling; 2: Vasocrine signaling

Figure: Role of WT in the development of atherosclerosis (25).

❖ **Quantification of epicardial adipose tissue:**

There is no consensus on how to measure WT. Three imaging methods have been proposed for WT quantification:

- **Ultrasound is the** simplest method of estimating epicardial fat. Ultrasound measurement of EAT thickness is performed via the left parasternal approach, anterior to the right cavities. The main shortcomings of this approach are that results are operator-dependent and quantification is only two-dimensional.
- **CT is** a relevant tool for quantifying WT thickness, as confirmed by the meta-analysis of Baohua Wu et al. The correlation between scannographic quantification of WT and coronary artery disease is based on evidence-based medicine (26). However, this now comes at the price of significant radiation exposure.
- **MRI is** the reference method for three-dimensional measurement of epicardial fat volume, thanks to its excellent contrast resolution: hypersignal adipose tissue in spin echo sequence, as well as in gradient echo. This is certainly a reliable, non-irradiating method, but it is long, costly and of limited availability in our country.

In this work, we chose transthoracic cardiac ultrasound as the means of assessing WT thickness. This choice was justified by new data in the literature arguing in favor of this imaging tool. Indeed, a recent meta-analysis evaluating WT thickness in coronary patients concluded that ultrasound measurement of WT appears to be an acceptable strategy for cardiovascular risk stratification, and that **ultrasound is the best means of WT assessment, combining** ease of use, absence of irradiation, accessibility and cost-effectiveness compared with other imaging modalities (27). A R Majumder et al had also confirmed the reliability of transthoracic ultrasound measurement of WT thickness for estimating coronary atherosclerosis, and that it could be used as a marker of coronary pathology (28).

- **WT: A new marker for coronary artery disease:**

Ectopic fats, such as WT and abdominal visceral fat, have been shown to be associated with increased cardiovascular events, independent of traditional risk factors (29). WT is increasingly attracting the attention of cardiovascular disease researchers.

The WT is currently identified as a new modifiable risk factor for the progression of atherosclerosis, and increased ultrasound thickness of the WT is an independent predictor of coronary disease risk(30), (27), (31).

Indeed, the meta-analysis published in 2018 had confirmed the evidence that sonographic WT thickness was increased in coronary patients and that the current challenge would be to determine the sonographic threshold of epicardial fat thickness at which a linear relationship with the risk of coronary artery disease exists(27). Furthermore, a study recently published in January 2022 by A RMajumder et al had suggested an echographic WT thickness>4.65mm as an independent predictor of significant coronary stenosis confirmed by coronary angiography(28).

The relationship between increased epicardial fat thickness and cardiovascular risk is complex and not fully elucidated. However, the dualism of the physiological and pathological effects of WT has been proposed as one of the substrates of this relationship.

Firstly, given the preferential pericoronary disposition of the WT, fat deposits around the myocardium and coronary arteries may play an important role in the pathogenesis of cardiovascular disease. Inflammatory and pro-atherogenic mediators secreted by the WT could intervene by diffusion into the interstitial fluid through the adventitia, or be transported through the vasa vasorum to the atherosclerotic plaque (Figure31).

This stimulation of vasa vasorum proliferation is responsible for structural alteration of the arterial wall (25).

But WT also secretes adipocytokines via its paracrine effect on the vascular wall of the coronary arteries. Mazurek et al showed that the WT of coronary patients was richer in macrophages, interleukins (IL) IL-1β and IL-6, and tumornecrosis factor-α (TNFa) than subcutaneous adipose tissue(5).WT overexpresses pro-inflammatory and pro-atherogenic factors including phospholipase sPLA2-IIA, angiotensinogen, plasminogen activator inhibitor, VascularEndothelialGrowth Factor (VEGF) and insulin-resistant adipokines such as resistin and visfatin(23). Phospholipase sPLA2-IIA appears to be present in atherosclerotic lesions and an independent factor in cardiovascular risk (32).

When inflammatory processes are activated, the epicardium becomes a site of altered adipogenesis. Adipocytes in the WT secrete pro-inflammatory adipokines and cytokines, with increased production of leptin and IL- 6 and decreased production of cardioprotective adiponectin leading to immune cell activation and inflammation, creating favorable conditions for the development and progression of atherosclerosis (24). Adipocytokines are involved in various processes, including inflammation, atrial and ventricular myocardial fibrosis and atherogenesis; and leptin is capable of affecting the vascular wall, activating platelet aggregation, thus increasing the risk of thrombosis. In addition, oxidative stress, macrophage activation and the inflammatory response induced by pro-inflammatory cytokines secreted by WT could induce atherogenic changes in monocytes and activation of endothelial adhesion, also implicated in the initiation of atherosclerosis by WT (33).

All in all, in the event of an inflammatory process, the WT is infiltrated by inflammatory cells, so the volume of the WT is increased. The status of adipokines and pro-inflammatory cytokines in WT adipocytes is altered, and they become overexpressed. Their secretion is increased, and these pro-inflammatory mediators are capable of inducing atherogenic changes in the vascular wall and the progression of coronary atherosclerosis.

11. Ultrasonographic assessment of WT thickness in patients and comparison with controls :

Median WT thickness was significantly higher in patients followed for SpA compared to healthy controls. Thus, it can be demonstrated that SpA patients are significantly more at risk of subclinical coronary atherosclerosis compared to healthy controls. Consequently, the SpA patients included had an increased cardiovascular risk, even though they were young patients (inclusion criterion: age ≤50 years) with a median age of 36 years, a predominant age range between 30 and 39 years, non-smokers and no known cardiovascular risk factors.This is a further argument in favour of the hypothesis that coronary atherosclerosis during SpA is accelerated by chronic inflammation in the absence of any cardiovascular risk factors.

Our results are in line with all the results available in the literature, which found a significantly higher WT thickness in SpA patients compared with controls. Table XXII summarizes the data from the various studies.

Sonographic assessment of epicardial fat in SpA has been little studied. To date, 8 studies have been carried out on this subject, and no meta-analysis is yet available. All were case-control studies evaluating the measurement of WT thickness by transthoracic cardiac echocardiography, and the number of SpA patients included ranged from 26 to 60. This is a further argument in favour of the representative number of our sample of 47 SpA patients without cardiovascular risk factors.

The median WT thickness in our patients was 3.1 mm (IQR 25-75%: 2.5-4). This was the lowest value compared with values found in other studies, which ranged from 4.35 mm to 7.3 mm. However, closer analysis of the patients' clinical and biological characteristics revealed that these patients were older (mean age between 38.6 and 46.6 years) versus 36 years in our sample (34), (35), (36), (37), (38), (39), (40).

Mean BMI was also higher than in our patients (34), (38), (40). On the other hand, patients included in these studies had higher values of lipid balance parameters (TC, LDL-C and TG) (34), (35), (36), (37), (41), (39), (40), smoking was not excluded in the studies by Demir et al (34), Çaglar et al (35), Surucu et al (41), Oz et al (40), Üstun et al (38) and Boyraz et al (39), and SpA was more active in 4 studies (34), (36), (41), (38).

Given that these parameters - age, smoking, BMI and lipid parameters - are known cardiovascular risk factors, they may explain why the WT thickness in our patients was lower, given the completeness of the selection criteria.

Table I: Results of the study of WT thickness in Spondyloarthritis in the literature.

	Number of SpA/Temoins	Average age of SpA patients (Years)	FRCV	SpA seniority (Years)	BMI (Kg/m)^2	Lipid balance (mg/dl)	CRP (mg/l)	ASDAS/ BASDAI	TAE SpA / Control thickness (mm)	p
Demir et al (2020) (34)	60/60	46,6 ± 8,7	Smoking not excluded	3 (1-7)	29,24 ± 5,11	C-HDL: 45.27 ± 9.54 C-LDL: 129.35± 27.03 TG: 152.94 ± 83.44	10 (3,3914,90)	NS / 4.10 ± 2.22	5,74 ±1,22/ 4,91 ± 1,21	<0,001
Çaglar et al (2016) (35)	42/40	39,3 ± 8,5	Tobacco +	NS	23,9±7,9	CT: 175 ± 38 TG: 124 ± 66	NS	NS / NS	7,3 ± 1,5 / 6,3 ± 0,7	<0,01
Resorlu et al(2014) (36)	40/40	42,7 ± 12,4	-	NS	24,7±3,6	HDL-C: 55.8 ± 17.4 C-LDL: 94.8 ± 12.8 TG: 101.05 ± 41,9	NS	NS / NS	4,35 ± 1,56/ 3,03 ± 0,94	<0,001

Büyükterzi et al (2019) (37)	50/50	39 (35-45)	-	NS	24,22 ± 3,11	CT: 208 (184224)C-HDL:46 (40- 54) C-LDL:138,5 (110150) TG: 132,50 (87170,5)	10,30 (3,3332,55)	NS / NS 48% had high activity according to ASDAS- CRP	4,75 (3,806,05) / 3,50 (3,104,00)	<0,001
Surucu el al (2018) (41)	38/38	35,42 ± 9,11	Smoking/dyslipidemia not excluded	3,5 ± 2,08	24,90 ± 1,82	CT: 185.21 ± 38.98 C-HDL: 44.79 ± 12.61 C-LDL: 108.89± 28.94 TG: 141.76 ± 93.37	9,9 ± 8,8	NS / 4.57 ± 1,84	4,5 ± 1,7/ 3,7 ± 1,0	0,01
Üstün et al (2014) (38)	26/26	43,7 ± 11,8	Tobacco +	11,83±10,98	28,1±5,3	NS	NS	NS / 4.2 ± 2,1	5,15± 1,13/ 4,11 ± 1,22	0,003
Boyraz et al (2016) (39)	30/25	38,6 ± 8,3	Smoking/dyslipidemia not excluded	8,8±8	25,18	CT: 174.8 ± 38.03 C-HDL: 47.8 ± 11.8 C-LDL: 99.76 ± 31.61 TG: 127.76 ± 62.95	NS	NS / 2.48 ± 2.21	NS: Higher value in SpA patients	NS

Oz et al (2020) (40)	43/42	42.8±9.2	Tobacco +	9.19±5.54	27.3 ± 4.9	CT: 194.7 ± 29.1 C-HDL: 47.9 ± 10.8 C-LDL: 122.8 ± 25.3 TG: 119.8 ± 61.1	7.28 ± 9.49	2,38 ± 0,**77/** 2,91 ± 1,86	4,6 ± 1,5 / 3,3 ± 1,2	<0,001

SpA: Spondyloarthritis; FRCV: cardiovascular risk factor; +: present; -:absent; BMI: body mass index; Kg: kilogram; m: metre; CRP: C-reactive protein; TAE: epicardial adipose tissue; mm: millimetre; ASDAS : Ankylosing Spondylitis Disease Activity Score; BASDAI: Bath Ankylosing Spondylitis Disease Activity Index; p: coefficient of significance; TC: total cholesterol; LDL: LDL cholesterol; HDL: HDL cholesterol; TG: triglycerides; NS: not specified.

12. Study of parameters influencing WT thickness in patients with Spondyloarthritis:

12.1 Patient parameters :

❖ **Age :**

Age was positively correlated with WT thickness, with low linearity. This was in line with the results reported in the literature. Resorlu et al (36) found a significant association between epicardial fat thickness and age in 40 patients with SpA and no cardiovascular comorbidities. Temiz et al (42) also confirmed this positive correlation between WT thickness and age in rheumatoid arthritis. Age is a known cardiovascular risk factor. Svanteson et al, investigating factors predictive of coronary risk in 86 rheumatic patients (rheumatoid arthritis, spondyloarthritis and psoriatic arthritis), concluded that age had the highest positive predictive value (43). Indeed, a study of adipokine expression in rats by Fei et al (44) showed that adiponectin expression by WT was significantly reduced with age.

This positive correlation in our results is important to consider. Despite the inclusion of young patients (≤ 50 years), age was
positively correlated with coronary atherosclerosis.

❖ **Blood pressure :**

Despite the non-inclusion of patients with arterial hypertension, we found a positive correlation between PAS levels and WT thickness. No association was found with diastolic blood pressure. Resorlu et al (36) found a significant association with diastolic blood pressure, with a trend towards significance for systolic blood pressure (p=0.05) in SpA.

The association between WT and blood pressure level was recently evaluated by a meta-analysis of the literature (45). WT thickness was significantly elevated in hypertensive patients. However, the pathophysiological mechanisms of this positive association remain poorly elucidated.

❖ **Anthropometric parameters :**

There was no significant association between WT thickness and the various anthropometric parameters studied. The positive relationship between WT and BMI

was found in the obese and in patients with metabolic syndrome (46), (47) . Interestingly, Gorter et al had noted that non-obese patients with multitruncular coronary disease had increased WT thickness.
(48) .

No significant association was found between anthropometric parameters and WT thickness during SpA(41), (37), (36).

5.1. Spondyloarthritis parameters :

- **Age of onset and duration of disease :**

WT thickness was positively correlated with age of disease onset, with a high predictive value in mutivariate analysis. Concerning the age of SpA, no correlation was found with WT thickness, unlike Surucu et al and Resorlu et al, who showed that WT thickness was significantly associated with the duration of disease progression in SpA (41), (36). This finding was verified in a cohort of 76 patients with rheumatoid arthritis (49). Thus, the development of atherosclerotic disease would be linked to the chronicity of the inflammatory process. The discrepancy with our result could be explained by the heterogeneity of the distribution of the age of SpA between patients.

- **Extra-articular manifestations:**

Patients with renal impairment had significantly higher WT thickness (p=0.05) with no significant correlation with creatinine levels (p=0.293). The association between cardiovascular risk and renal function is widely recognized. Indeed, cardiovascular complications are the 1ère cause of cardiovascular morbidity and mortality in patients with chronic renal failure(50). However, the association between WT and renal impairment has not been studied in the literature. A study by Reinhardt et al (51) in young patients with type 2 diabetes showed that WT thickness was significantly associated with glomerular filtration rate (GFR) and was predictive of impaired renal function.

Larger-scale studies are needed to investigate the relationship between WT and renal impairment in SpA.

- **Pain :**

WT thickness was positively correlated with overall pain VAS and BASG-s score in a statistically significant manner.

Studying carotid intima-media thickness as a screening marker for sub-clinical atherosclerosis in SpA(52), Hamdi et al found, in line with our results, a significant positive association between global spinal pain VAS and carotid intima-media thickness. However, the influence of PROs on WT thickness in SpA has not been studied in the literature.

- **Disease activity :**

In our patients, no significant association was found between epicardial fat thickness and inflammation parameters, namely disease activity scores (ASDAS-CRP and BASDAI) and CRP levels. Ustün et al (38), Surucu et al (41), Resorlu et al (36) found no significant association between WT thickness and SpA activity scores, CRP or sedimentation rate.

In contrast, in the study by Büyükterzi et al (37) of 50 SpA patients without cardiovascular comorbidities, the ASDAS-CRP score was significantly related to WT thickness ($p<0.001$), with a strong positive predictive value in multivariate analysis. This could be explained by the fluctuating inflammatory state over time and its modification by disease-modifying treatments.

- **Spine metrology:**

A significant negative correlation was found between WT thickness and dorsal spine involvement as assessed by thoracic ampliation. Thus, dorsal stiffness was associated with increased epicardial fat thickness. This association has not been studied in the literature. Thoracic ampliation was inversely correlated with ultrasound measurement of carotid intima-media thickness, a validated parameter for the assessment of sub-clinical atherosclerosis in a Tunisian and Hungarian population (52), (53).in accordance with the study by Ustün et al (38), no significant correlation was found between epicardial fat thickness and BASMI score. Further large-scale studies are needed to investigate the influence of spinal mobility on EAT thickness.

- **Functional impact**

As regards the BASFI score, no significant association was found. Among the results available in the literature, 2 studies were in agreement with our results (36), (38) and a third study showed a positive association between WT thickness and BASFI score in SpA (41).

- **Structural damage :**

Structural damage was significantly associated with the risk of coronary atherosclerosis in our SpA patients. Indeed, we found that WT thickness was significantly higher in patients with syndesmophytes, intervertebral bone bridges or posterior joint involvement. Moreover, WT thickness was positively correlated with mSASSS score. In multivariate analysis, the mSASSS score was the strongest predictor: each unit increase in mSASSS increased epicardial fat thickness by 0.064 mm.

The relationship between WT thickness and spinal structural damage in SpA has not been studied in the literature. To our knowledge, this is the first study to show a positive association between structural damage and epicardial fat thickness. Recently published data have suggested a link between structural damage in SpA (syndesmophytes, bone bridges, mSASSS score) and accelerated atherosclerosis as assessed by progression of carotid intima-media thickness (54), (55).

Kang et al (56), in their study of a cohort of 185 patients with axial SpA and no known cardiovascular risk factors, showed that the number of syndesmophytes was independently associated with the Framingham score estimating coronary risk within 10 years.

- **Therapeutic modalities :**

- **Non-steroidal anti-inflammatory drugs :**

There was no significant difference in WT thickness according to the type of NSAID prescribed (p=0.081). There was no correlation with NSAID consumption as assessed by the ASAS-NSAID index (p=0.90).

The influence of non-steroidal anti-inflammatory drugs (NSAIDs) on WT has not been studied in the literature. However, the increased risk of cardiovascular events, as well as a disturbance in blood pressure balance, under NSAIDs has been widely reported (57). Median WT thickness was highest in patients on anti-COX2, with no significant difference. This deleterious role of selective NSAIDs in excess cardiovascular risk has been highlighted in the literature, with anti-COX2s associated with elevated cardiovascular risk (58), (59).

- **Anti-TNF alpha :**

Median WT thickness was significantly higher in our anti-TNF alpha-treated patients (3.95mm versus 2.7mm in biotherapy-naive patients). The influence of anti-TNF alpha on WT in SpA has not yet been studied in the literature. There is a single study evaluating the effect of anti-TNF alpha on WT thickness in rheumatoid arthritis, whose findings argued in favour of a vascular protective effect of anti - TNF (60); WT thickness was significantly reduced in patients treated with anti-TNF alpha compared with patients treated with csDMARDS (p = 0.04).

The protective role of anti-TNF alpha via its anti-inflammatory effect has been reported in the literature, but remains controversial. Indeed, the markers of sub-clinical atherosclerosis studied were FMD for endothelial dysfunction, carotid intima-media thickness and arterial stiffness markers. Although some studies concluded that anti-TNF alpha had a positive effect, with a reduction in carotid intima-media thickness (61), (62) or an improvement in endothelial dysfunction and arterial stiffness (63) in SpA treated with anti-TNF alpha as opposed to biologically naïve patients, other series did not support this hypothesis and showed no improvement in intima-media thickness or its progression with anti-TNF alpha (64), (65).

A recent meta-analysis reviewing the effect of anti-TNF alpha on markers of atherosclerosis in chronic inflammatory rheumatism found no strong evidence for a confirmed positive vascular protective effect of anti-TNF alpha (66).

The small size and heterogeneity of our population, as well as the median age and duration of disease progression, which were significantly higher in patients treated with anti-TNF alpha (43 years and 12 years respectively) than in the biotherapy-naive group (32 years and 7 years respectively,($p<0.009$ and <0.004), do not allow us to conclude that anti-TNF alpha has a negative cardiovascular effect. Larger-scale studies on the influence of anti-TNF alpha on WT are needed.

5.2. Biological data :

- **Fasting blood glucose:**

We found no significant correlation between WT thickness and fasting blood glucose, in line with studies that have investigated factors associated with elevated epicardial fat in SpA (36), (37). This could be explained by the selection criteria of our population; all subjects had normal fasting blood glucose levels with the exception of one patient who had fasting blood glucose at the upper limit (5.91 mmol/l). Aydin et al (67) and Iacobellis et al(68)showed that WT thickness was significantly correlated with fasting blood glucose in patients with metabolic syndrome. This seems logical, given that metabolic syndrome is associated with cardiovascular risk.

- **Lipid balance:**

There was a significant positive correlation between WT thickness and triglyceridemia, with low linearity. In multivariate analysis, triglyceride level was a strong predictor of WT thickness: each 1 unit increase in triglyceridemia increased epicardial fat thickness by 0.661 mm. WT is thought to be characterized by its high triglyceride content (25) and its capacity to release free fatty acids into the coronary circulation as a source of energy.

This result is perfectly explained by the pathophysiology of ectopic fat. We recall that the initial anomaly responsible for the development of ectopic fat is a dysfunction of the subcutaneous adipose tissue, which no longer plays its protective role as a metabolic purifier, either because it is unable to develop (lipodystrophy), or because it has become hypertrophic, dysfunctional and insulin-resistant. The dysfunction of subcutaneous adipose tissue, combined with the development of visceral adipose tissue secreting pro-inflammatory factors, is thought to promote ectopy (69).

Adipose tissue responds to metabolic stress with increased secretion of pro-inflammatory molecules with local and systemic action, strongly correlated with insulin resistance. Insulin resistance is thus a consequence of ectopic lipid storage. Muscular insulin resistance promotes the muscle's inability to control mitochondrial fatty acid oxidation properly, with preferential orientation of carbohydrate oxidation from muscle to liver, which stimulates de novo lipogenesis and hepatic triglyceride production (70). Thus, the development of WT is associated with the accumulation of triglycerides outside adipose tissue.

The study by Resorlu et al (36) reinforces our findings. They also found a significant positive association between WT thickness and triglyceridemia in 40 SpA patients with no cardiovascular risk factors.

There was no association with levels of TC, LDL-C, HDL-C or the TC/HDL-C and LDL-C/HDL ratios. Our results were in line with those published by Büyükterzi et al (37) and Resorlu et al (36). However, Surucu et al (41) found a statistically significant negative association between WT thickness and TC (p=0.016; r=-0.276) and LDL-C (p=0.009; r :-0.299) in patients with SpA.

- **CRP:**

No significant correlation was found between CRP and WT thickness. This result was in agreement with other authors (37), (41). The median CRP in our patients was 6.45 mg/l, and this relatively low level may explain the lack of a significant relationship between this serum marker of inflammation and WT thickness.

Table: Factors associated with WT thickness in patients with SpA in the literature.

Study	Patient parameters	p	SpA-related parameters	p
Resorlu et al (36)	Age PAD Triglyceridemia	0,001 0,041 0.011	Age of SpA	0,002
Surucu et al (41)	CT C-LDL	0,016 0,009	Age of SpA BASFI	0,012 0,008
Büyükterzi and a (37)	Not association significant	-	ASDAS-CRP	<0,001
Çaglar et al (35)	NE	-	NE	-
Boyraz et al (39)	NE	-	NE	-
Demir et al (34)	NE	-	NE	-

Ustün et al (38)	NE	-	No significant association	-
Oz et al (40)	NE	-	NE	-

NE: Not studied; p: coefficient of significance; SpA: spondyloarthritis; PAD: diastolic blood pressure; CRP: reactive protein-C; ASDAS: Ankylosing spondylitis disease activity score.

13. Predictive factors - Multivariate analysis :

The independent predictors of increased WT thickness associated with accelerated coronary atherosclerosis identified were: age of SpA onset, mSASSS score and TG level. The mSASSS score was the strongest predictor.

Triglyceridemia is a well-known traditional cardiovascular risk factor. This underlines the importance of monitoring lipid status even in young SpA patients with no cardiovascular risk factors. The other two factors predictive of coronary atherosclerosis were disease-related parameters. To our knowledge, this is the first study to identify radiographic mSASSS score as a predictor of increased epicardial fat thickness in SpA.

This supports and confirms that chronic inflammation in SpA is the most important parameter in the acceleration of atherosclerosis in these patients. Hence the importance of intensive management of patients with SpA, even those consulting at a late stage with proven structural damage.

Chapter 3

14. Recommendations - Prospects :

Young SpA patients (≤50 years of age) free of any cardiovascular risk factors or comorbidities had significantly higher WT thickness than age-, sex- and BMI-matched control subjects. Thus, these young SpAs with low disease activity have a greater risk of coronary atherosclerosis than the general population.

This marker of sub-clinical atherosclerosis has been proposed as an independent predictor of CHD risk, and can be used for cardiovascular risk stratification. However, larger-scale multicenter studies are needed.

We propose the following recommendations:

- ➢ Identify theSpA patient at high coronary risk if he presents at least :
  - ■ Advanced age of onset of SpA.
  - ■ A traditional cardiovascular risk factor: high systolic blood pressure, hypertriglyceridemia.
  - ■ Extra-articular renal involvement.
  - ■ Spinal structural damage.
- ➢ Annual screening for conventional cardiovascular risk factors on a regular basis in collaboration with cardiologists:
  - ■ Annual blood pressure measurement.
  - ■ Monitor lipid and creatinine levels.
- ➢ Management of traditional cardiovascular risk factors and cardiovascular comorbidities :

  Balancing diabetes, hypertension and dyslipidemia is an essential step in primary prevention.

  - ■ Diabetes: prescription of thiazolidinedione-type antidiabetics, glucagon-like peptide-1 (GLP-1) analogue or DPP-4 inhibitor in type 2 diabetic patients was associated with a significant reduction in WT thickness and attenuation of its inflammatory profile (71).
  - ■ Combating sedentary lifestyles and promoting a program of regular physical activity: studies have shown a significant reduction in WT thickness after a

program of regular aerobic exercise (57), (58), (59) The response of WT was greater and faster than that of other adipose tissues.

- Management of obesity and overweight: weight-reduction procedures using bariatric surgery have shown a significant and rapid reduction in WT thickness(72),(73),(74),(75).

- Encourage a Mediterranean-style diet in line with HAS recommendations, with more unsaturated fatty acids and less saturated fatty acids:

  A comparative experimental study conducted in 2019 by Walker et al (76)demonstrated that the polyunsaturated fatty acid diet was associated with significant expression of anti-inflammatory signaling genes by the WT (PPARG, FFAR4 and ADIPOQ). In contrast, pigs on the saturated fatty acid diet expressed more inflammatory signaling genes.

- Discuss the prescription of statins in the presence of risk factors (hypertriglyceridemia, TAE hypertrophy):

  A significant reduction in WT thickness has been reported with statins, particularly atorvastatin (77), (78). This reduction was uncorrelated with improvement in lipid balance parameters, suggesting an independent pharmacological effect of statins on WT.At the conclusion of this work; we concluded that young SpA patients without FRCV have an increased risk of atherosclerosis compared with the general population. Epicardial fat thickness is an independent predictor of coronary artery disease. Ultrasound measurement of epicardial fat is simple, rapid, accessible, reliable and non-irradiating. Thus, this tool can be used in clinical practice as a means of screening for sub-clinical atherosclerosis. We therefore propose to establish a consensus in collaboration with cardiologists and to validate it through a multicenter study and an expert committee in order to improve the vital prognosis of our young rheumatic patients.

Conclusion

SpA is the second most common chronic inflammatory rheumatic disease, preferentially affecting young male subjects. Despite major advances in SpA treatment, the 1ère cause of death is cardiovascular. This increase in cardiovascular morbidity and mortality is secondary to atherosclerosis accelerated by chronic inflammation.

However, evaluation methods

References :

1. Wendling D, Lukas C, Paccou J, Claudepierre P, Carton L, Combe B, et al. Recommendations of the french society for rheumatology (SFR) on the everyday management of patients with spondyloarthritis. Joint Bone Spine. 2014;81(1):6-14.

2. Toussirot E. The risk of cardiovascular diseases in axial spondyloarthritis. Current Insights. Front Med. 2021;8:782150.

3. Prati C, Demougeot C, Guillot X, Sondag M, Verhoeven F, Wendling D. Atteinte of vessels in axial spondyloarthritis. Rev Rhum. 2018;85(5):448- 52.

4. Yuan Y, Yang J, Zhang X, Han R, Chen M, Hu X, et al. Carotid intima-media thickness in patients with ankylosing spondylitis: a systematic review and updated meta-analysis. J Atheroscler Thromb. 2019;26(3):260-71.

5. Bai R, Zhang Y, Liu W, Ma C, Chen X, Yang J, et al. The relationship of ankylosing spondylitis and subclinical atherosclerosis: a systemic review and metaanalysis. Angiology. 2019;70(6):492-500.

6. Hatipsoylu E, Çengül Í, Kaya T, Karatepe AG, Akçay S, Isayeva L, et al. Assessment of subclinical atherosclerotic cardiovascular disease in patients with ankylosing spondylitis. Anatol J Cardiol. 2019;22(4):185-91.

7. Kaplanoglu H, Ozi⅞ler C. Evaluation of subclinical atherosclerosis using ultrasound. radiofrequency data technology in patients diagnosed with ankylosing spondylitis: evaluation of subclinical atherosclerosis in ankylosing spondylitis. J Ultrasound Med. 2019;38(3):703-11.

8. González Mazón I, Rueda Gotor J, Ferraz Amaro I, Genre F, Corrales A, Calvo Rio V, et al. Subclinical atherosclerotic disease in ankylosing spondylitis and nonradiographic axial spondyloarthritis. A multicenter study on 806 patients. Semin Arthritis Rheum. 2021;51(2):395-403.

9. Kerekes G, Soltész P, Nurmohamed MT, Gonzalez Gay MA, Turiel M, Végh E, et al. Validated methods for assessment of subclinical atherosclerosis in

rheumatology. Nat Rev Rheumatol. 2012;8(4):224-34.

10. Moroni L, Selmi C, Angelini C, Meroni PL. Evaluation of endothelial function by flow-mediated dilation: a comprehensive review in rheumatic disease. Arch Immunol Ther Exp. 2017;65(6):463-75.

11. Losinska K, Korkosz M, Kwasny Krochin B. Endothelial dysfunction in patients with ankylosing spondylitis. Reumatologia. 2019;57(2):100-5.

12. Godo S, Shimokawa H. Endothelial functions. Arterioscler Thromb Vasc Biol. 2017;37(9):108-14.

13. Cyr AR, Huckaby LV, Shiva SS, Zuckerbraun BS. Nitric oxide and endothelial dysfunction. Crit Care Clin. 2020;36(2):307-21.

14. Bugnard IL, Rangueil C. Endothelial dysfunction and atherosclerosis [Online]. Réalités Cardiologiques [cited 14/11/2021]; [7 pages]. Available from URL: https://www.realites-cardiologiques.com/wp-content/uploads/sites/2/2011/01/112.pdf

15. Shimbo D, Grahame Clarke C, Miyake Y, Rodriguez C, Sciacca R, Di Tullio M, et al. al. The association between endothelial dysfunction and cardiovascular outcomes in a population-based multi-ethnic cohort. Atherosclerosis. 2007;192(1):197-203.

16. Puissant C, Abraham P, Durand S, Humeau Heurtier A, Faure S, Rousseau P, et al. Endothelial function: role, assessment methods and limitations. J Mal Vasc. 2014;39(1):47-56.

17. Celermajer DS. Reliable endothelial function testing: at our fingertips? Circulation. 2008;117(19):2428-30.

18. Vogiatzi G, Tousoulis D, Stefanadis C. The role of oxidative stress in atherosclerosis. Hellenic J Cardiol. 2009;50(5):402-9.

19. Stanek A, Cholewka A, Wielkoszynski T, Romuk E, Sieron K, Sieron A. Increased levels of oxidative stress markers, soluble CD40 ligand, and carotid intimamedia thickness reflect acceleration of atherosclerosis in male patients with ankylosing spondylitis in active phase and without the classical cardiovascular risk factors.

Oxid Med Cell Longev. 2017;2017:9712536.

20. Gach O, Piérard L, Legrand V. Inflammation and atherosclerosis: state of the art question in 2004-2005. Rev Med Liege. 2005;60(4):235-41.

21. Zhu Y, Xian X, Wang Z, Bi Y, Chen Q, Han X, et al. Research progress on the relationship between atherosclerosis and inflammation. Biomolecules. 2018;8(3):80.

22. Willeit P, Tschiderer L, Allara E, Reuber K, Seekircher L, Gao L, et al. Carotid intima-media thickness progression as surrogate marker for cardiovascular risk: meta-analysis of 119 clinical trials involving 100 667 patients. Circulation. 2020;142(7):621-42.

23. Kavurma MM, Rayner KJ, Karunakaran D. The walking dead: macrophage inflammation and death in atherosclerosis. Curr Opin Lipidol. 2017;28(2):91-8 .

24. Criqui MH, Denenberg JO, Bird CE, Fronek A, Klauber MR, Langer RD. The correlation between symptoms and non-invasive test results in patients referred for peripheral arterial disease testing. Vasc Med. 1996;1(1):65-71.

25. Ankle Brachial Index Collaboration. Ankle brachial index combined with framingham risk score to predict cardiovascular events and mortality: a metaanalysis. J Am Med Assoc. 2008;300(2):197-208.

26. Bakland G, Gran JT, Nossent JC. Increased mortality in ankylosing spondylitis is related to disease activity. Ann Rheum Dis. 2011;70(11):1921-5.

27. Liew JW, Ramiro S, Gensler LS. Cardiovascular morbidity and mortality in ankylosing spondylitis and psoriatic arthritis. Best Pract Res Clin Rheumatol. 2018;32(3):369-89.

28. Prati C, Claudepierre P, Pham T, Wendling D. Mortality in spondylarthritis. Joint Bone Spine. 2011;78(5):466-70.

29. Castaneda S, Nurmohamed MT, González Gay MA. Cardiovascular disease in inflammatory rheumatic diseases. Best Pract Res Clin Rheumatol.

2016;30(5):851-69.

30. Mathieu S, Soubrier M. Cardiovascular risk in spondyloarthritis. axial. Presse Med. 2015;44(9):907-11.

31. Peters ML, Visman I, Nielen MJ, Van Dillen N, Verheij RA, Van Der Horst Bruinsma IE, et al. Ankylosing spondylitis: a risk factor for myocardial infarction: table 1. Ann Rheum Dis. 2010;69(3):579-81.

32. Eriksson JK, Jacobsson L, Bengtsson K, Askling J. Is ankylosing spondylitis a risk factor for cardiovascular disease, and how do these risks compare with those in rheumatoid arthritis? Ann Rheum Dis. 2017;76(2):364-70.

33. Huang YP, Wang YH, Pan SL. Increased risk of ischemic heart disease in young patients with newly diagnosed ankylosing spondylitis - a population-based longitudinal follow-up study. PLoS One. 2013;8(5):e64155.

34. Brophy S, Cooksey R, Atkinson M, Zhou SM, Husain MJ, Macey S, et al. No increased rate of acute myocardial infarction or stroke among patients with ankylosing spondylitis-a retrospective cohort study using routine data. Semin Arthritis Rheum. 2012;42(2):140-5.

35. Bosmans LA, Bosch L, Kusters PH, Lutgens E, Seijkens TP. The CD40-CD40L dyad as immunotherapeutic target in cardiovascular disease. J Cardiovasc Transl Res. 2021;14(1):13-22.

36. Arida A, Protogerou AD, Konstantonis G, Konsta M, Delicha EM, Kitas GD, et al. Subclinical atherosclerosis is not accelerated in patients with ankylosing spondylitis with low disease activity: new data and metaanalysis of published studies. J Rheumatol. 2015;42(11):2098-105.

37. Kucuk A, Ugur Uslu A, Icli A, Cure E, Arslan S, Turkmen K, et al. The LDL/HDL ratio and atherosclerosis in ankylosing spondylitis. Z Rheumatol. 2017;76(1):58-63.

38. Choe JY, Lee MY, Rheem I, Rhee MY, Park SH, Kim SK. No differences of carotid intima-media thickness between young patients with ankylosing spondylitis and

healthy controls. Joint Bone Spine. 2008;75(5):548-53.

39. Cure E, Icli A, Uslu AU, Sakiz D, Cure MC, Baykara RA, et al. Atherogenic index of plasma: a useful marker for subclinical atherosclerosis in ankylosing spondylitis: AIP associate with cIMT in AS. Clin Rheumatol. 2018;37(5):1273-80.

40. Ladehesa Pineda ML, Arias De La Rosa I, López Medina C, Castro Villegas MC, Ábalos Aguilera MC, Ortega Castro R, et al. Assessment of the relationship between estimated cardiovascular risk and structural damage in patients with axial spondyloarthritis. Ther Adv Musculoskelet Dis. 2020;12:1759720X20982837.

41. Rueda Gotor J, Quevedo Abeledo JC, Corrales A, Genre F, Hernández Hernández V, Delgado Frías E, et al. Reclassification into very-high cardiovascular risk after carotid ultrasound in patients with axial spondyloarthritis. Clin Exp Rheumatol. 2020;38(4):724-31.

42. Serdaroglu Beyazal M, Erdogan T, Türkyilmaz AK, Devrimsel G, Cüre MC, Beyazal M, et al. Relationship of serum osteoprotegerin with arterial stiffness, preclinical atherosclerosis, and disease activity in patients with ankylosing spondylitis. Clin Rheumatol. 2016;35(9):2235-41.

43. Resorlu H, Akbal A, Resorlu M, Gokmen F, Ates C, Uysal F, et al. Epicardial adipose tissue thickness in patients with ankylosing spondylitis. Clin Rheumatol. 2015;34(2):295-9.

44. Hamdi W, Chelli Bouaziz M, Zouch I, Ghannouchi MM, Haouel M, Ladeb MF, et al. Assessment of preclinical atherosclerosis in patients with ankylosing spondylitis. J Rheumatol. 2012;39(2):322-6.

45. Giollo A, Dalbeni A, Cioffi G, Ognibeni F, Gatti D, Idolazzi L, et al. Factors associated with accelerated subclinical atherosclerosis in patients with spondyloarthritis without overt cardiovascular disease. Clin Rheumatol. 2017;36(11):2487-95.

46. Perrotta FM, Scarno A, Carboni A, Bernardo V, Montepaone M, Lubrano E, et al. Assessment of subclinical atherosclerosis in ankylosing spondylitis: correlations with disease activity indices. Reumatismo. 2013;65(3):105-12.

47. Singh T, Newman AB. Inflammatory markers in population studies of aging. Ageing Res Rev. 2011;10(3):319-29.

48. Gonzalez Juanatey C, Vazquez Rodriguez TR, Miranda Filloy JA, Dierssen T, Vaqueiro I, Blanco R, et al. The high prevalence of subclinical atherosclerosis in patients with ankylosing spondylitis without clinically evident cardiovascular disease. Medicine. 2009;88(6):358-65.

49. Sari I, Okan T, Akar S, Cece H, Altay C, Secil M, et al. Impaired endothelial function in patients with ankylosing spondylitis. Rheumatology. 2006;45(3):283-6.

50. Verma I, Syngle A, Krishan P, Garg N. Endothelial progenitor cells as a marker of endothelial dysfunction and atherosclerosis in ankylosing spondylitis: a cross-sectional study. Int J Angiol. 2016;26(01):036-42.

51. Bodnár N, Kerekes G, Seres I, Paragh G, Kappelmayer J, Némethné ZG, et al. Assessment of subclinical vascular disease associated with ankylosing spondylitis. J Rheumatol. 2011;38(4):723-9.

52. Erre GL, Mangoni AA, Castagna F, Paliogiannis P, Carru C, Passiu G, et al. Meta Analysis of asymmetric dimethylarginine concentrations in rheumatic diseases. Sci Rep. 2019;9:5426.

53. Berg IJ, Van Der Heijde D, Dagfinrud H, Seljeflot I, Olsen IC, Kvien TK, et al. Disease activity in ankylosing spondylitis and associations to markers of vascular pathology and traditional cardiovascular disease risk factors: a cross-sectional study. J Rheumatol. 2015;42(4):645-53.

54. Przepiera Bqdzak H, Fischer K, Brzosko M. Serum interleukin-18, fetuin-a, soluble intercellular adhesion molecule-1, and endothelin-1 in ankylosing spondylitis, psoriatic arthritis, and SAPHO syndrome. Int J Mol Sci. 2016;17(8):1255.

1. Wendling D, Lukas C, Paccou J, Claudepierre P, Carton L, Combe B, et al. Recommendations of the french society for rheumatology (SFR) on the everyday management of patients with spondyloarthritis. Joint Bone Spine. 2014;81(1):6-14.

2. Toussirot E. The risk of cardiovascular diseases in axial spondyloarthritis. Current Insights. Front Med. 2021;8:782150.

3. Prati C, Demougeot C, Guillot X, Sondag M, Verhoeven F, Wendling D. Atteinte of vessels in axial spondyloarthritis. Rev Rhum. 2018;85(5):448- 52.

4. Yuan Y, Yang J, Zhang X, Han R, Chen M, Hu X, et al. Carotid intima-media thickness in patients with ankylosing spondylitis: a systematic review and updated meta-analysis. J Atheroscler Thromb. 2019;26(3):260-71.

5. Bai R, Zhang Y, Liu W, Ma C, Chen X, Yang J, et al. The relationship of ankylosing spondylitis and subclinical atherosclerosis: a systemic review and metaanalysis.Angiology. 2019;70(6):492-500.

6. Hatipsoylu E, Çengül Í, Kaya T, Karatepe AG, Akçay S, Isayeva L, et al. Assessment of subclinical atherosclerotic cardiovascular disease in patients with ankylosing spondylitis. Anatol J Cardiol. 2019;22(4):185-91.

7. Kaplanoglu H, Ozi⅞ler C. Evaluation of subclinical atherosclerosis using ultrasound. radiofrequency data technology in patients diagnosed with ankylosing spondylitis: evaluation of subclinical atherosclerosis in ankylosing spondylitis. J Ultrasound Med. 2019;38(3):703-11.

8. González Mazón I, Rueda Gotor J, Ferraz Amaro I, Genre F, Corrales A, Calvo Rio V, et al. Subclinical atherosclerotic disease in ankylosing spondylitis and nonradiographic axial spondyloarthritis. A multicenter study on 806 patients. Semin Arthritis Rheum. 2021;51(2):395-403.

9. Kerekes G, Soltész P, Nurmohamed MT, Gonzalez Gay MA, Turiel M, Végh E, et al. Validated methods for assessment of subclinical atherosclerosis in rheumatology. Nat Rev Rheumatol. 2012;8(4):224-34.

10. Moroni L, Selmi C, Angelini C, Meroni PL. Evaluation of endothelial function by flow-mediated dilation: a comprehensive review in rheumatic disease. Arch Immunol Ther Exp. 2017;65(6):463-75.

11. Rudwaleit M, Van Der Heijde D, Landewe R, Listing J, Akkoc N, Brandt J, et al. The development of assessment of spondyloarthritis international society classification criteria for axial spondyloarthritis (part II): validation and final selection. Ann Rheum Dis. 2009;68(6):777-83.

12. Kemta Lekpa F, Claudepierre P. Spondyloarthritis, from diagnosis to nosology: criteria and limits. Revue du Rhumatisme Monographies. 2014;81(4):218-24.

13. Jones SD, Steiner A, Garrett SL, Calin A. The bath ankylosing spondylitis patient global score (BAS-G). Rheumatology. 1996;35(1):66-71.

14. Chilton Mitchell L, Martindale J, Hart A, Goodacre L. Normative values for the bath ankylosing spondylitis metrology index in a UK population. Rheumatology. 2013;52(11):2086-90.

15. Heuft-Dorenbosch L, Spoorenberg A, van Tubergen A, Landewe R, van ver Tempel H, Mielants H, et al. Assessment of enthesitis in ankylosing spondylitis. Ann Rheum Dis 2003; **62**: 127-32.

16. Garrett S, Jenkinson T, Kennedy LG, Whitelock H, Gaisford P, Calin A. A new approach to defining disease status in ankylosing spondylitis: the Bath Ankylosing Spondylitis Disease Activity Index. J Rheumatol 1994; 21:2286-91

17. Kchir MM, Hamdi W, Kochbati S, Azzouz D, Daoud L, Saadellaoui K, et al. Validation of the Tunisian versions of bath ankylosing spondylitis functional index (BASFI) and disease activity index (BASDAI). Tunis Med. 2009;87(8):527-30.

18. Lukas C, Landewé R, Sieper J, Dougados M, Davis J, Braun J, et al. Development of an ASAS-endorsed disease activity score (ASDAS) in patients with ankylosing spondylitis. Ann Rheum Dis. 2009;68(1):18-24.

19. Lequesne M. Indices of severity and disease activity for osteoarthritis. Semin Arthritis Rheum. 1991;20(2):48-54.

20. MacKay K, Mack C, Brophy S, Calin A. The bath ankylosing spondylitis radiology index (BASRI): a new, validated approach to disease assessment. Arthritis Rheum. 1998;41(12):2263-70.

21. Llop M, Rios Rodriguez V, Redeker I, Sieper J, Haibel H, Rudwaleit M, et al. Incorporation of the anteroposterior lumbar radiographs in the modified stoke ankylosing spondylitis spine score improves detection of radiographic spinal progression in axial spondyloarthritis. Arthritis Res Ther. 2019;21(1):126.

22. P Louyot,G Jung,J Pourel, J R Graff,Y Montet. [Coxitis in ankylosing spondylarthritis]. Rev Rhum Mal Osteoartic. 1970;37(1):19-41

23. Mendonça JA, Bisetto De Andrade B, Braga De Aquino JL, Leandro Merhi VA, Damian GB. Spectral doppler and automated software-guided ultrasound assessment of bilateral common carotid intima-media thickness in spondyloarthritis: is there a correlation with clinical findings? Drugs Context. 2018;7:212538.

24. Choi H, Uceda DE, Dey AK, Mehta NN. Application of non-invasive imaging in inflammatory disease conditions to evaluate subclinical coronary artery disease. Curr Rheumatol Rep. 2020;22(1):1.

25. Thijssen DJ, Bruno RM, Van Mil AM, Holder SM, Faita F, Greyling A, et al. Expert consensus and evidence-based recommendations for the assessment of flow-mediated dilation in humans. Eur Heart J. 2019;40(30):2534-47.

26. Lima BB, Quyyumi AA, Vaccarino V. A future for flow-mediated dilation-just follow the guidelines-reply. JAMA Cardiol. 2020;5(3):361.

27. Harris RA, Nishiyama SK, Wray DW, Richardson RS. Ultrasound assessment of flow-mediated dilation. Hypertension. 2010;55(5):1075-85.

28. Aboyans V, Criqui MH, Abraham P, Allison MA, Creager MA, Diehm C, et al. Measurement and interpretation of the ankle-brachial index: a scientific statement from the american heart association. Circulation. 2012;126(24):2890-

909.

29. Hiatt WR. Medical treatment of peripheral arterial disease and claudication. N Engl J Med. 2001;344(21):1608-21.

30. Abdessalem S, Majadlah S, Bouslimi N, Mourali S, Mechemeche R. The study of endothelial function predicts the existence and severity of coronary artery disease.Tunis Med. 2009;87(12):843-50.

31. Losinska K, Korkosz M, Kwasny Krochin B. Endothelial dysfunction in patients with ankylosing spondylitis. Reumatologia. 2019;57(2):100-5.

32. Godo S, Shimokawa H. Endothelial functions. Arterioscler Thromb Vasc Biol. 2017;37(9):108-14.

33. Cyr AR, Huckaby LV, Shiva SS, Zuckerbraun BS. Nitric oxide and endothelial dysfunction. Crit Care Clin. 2020;36(2):307-21.

34. Bugnard IL, Rangueil C. Endothelial dysfunction and atherosclerosis [Online]. Réalités Cardiologiques [cited 14/11/2021]; [7 pages]. Available from URL: https://www.realites-cardiologiques.com/wp-content/uploads/sites/2/2011/01/112.pdf

35. Shimbo D, Grahame Clarke C, Miyake Y, Rodriguez C, Sciacca R, Di Tullio M, et al. al. The association between endothelial dysfunction and cardiovascular outcomes in a population-based multi-ethnic cohort. Atherosclerosis. 2007;192(1):197-203.

36. Puissant C, Abraham P, Durand S, Humeau Heurtier A, Faure S, Rousseau P, et al. Endothelial function: role, assessment methods and limitations. J Mal Vasc. 2014;39(1):47-56.

37. Celermajer DS. Reliable endothelial function testing: at our fingertips? Circulation. 2008;117(19):2428-30.

38. Vogiatzi G, Tousoulis D, Stefanadis C. The role of oxidative stress in atherosclerosis. Hellenic J Cardiol. 2009;50(5):402-9.

39. Stanek A, Cholewka A, Wielkoszynski T, Romuk E, Sieron K, Sieron A. Increased levels of oxidative stress markers, soluble CD40 ligand, and carotid intimamedia thickness reflect acceleration of atherosclerosis in male patients with ankylosing spondylitis in active phase and without the classical cardiovascular risk factors. Oxid Med Cell Longev. 2017;2017:9712536.

40. Gach O, Piérard L, Legrand V. Inflammation and atherosclerosis: state of the art question in 2004-2005. Rev Med Liege. 2005;60(4):235-41.

41. Zhu Y, Xian X, Wang Z, Bi Y, Chen Q, Han X, et al. Research progress on the relationship between atherosclerosis and inflammation. Biomolecules. 2018;8(3):80.

42. Willeit P, Tschiderer L, Allara E, Reuber K, Seekircher L, Gao L, et al. Carotid intima-media thickness progression as surrogate marker for cardiovascular risk: meta-analysis of 119 clinical trials involving 100 667 patients. Circulation. 2020;142(7):621-42.

43. Kavurma MM, Rayner KJ, Karunakaran D. The walking dead: macrophage inflammation and death in atherosclerosis. Curr Opin Lipidol. 2017;28(2):91- 8.

44. Criqui MH, Denenberg JO, Bird CE, Fronek A, Klauber MR, Langer RD. The correlation between symptoms and non-invasive test results in patients referred for peripheral arterial disease testing. Vasc Med. 1996;1(1):65-71.

45. Ankle Brachial Index Collaboration. Ankle brachial index combined with framingham risk score to predict cardiovascular events and mortality: a metaanalysis. J Am Med Assoc. 2008;300(2):197-208.

46. Bakland G, Gran JT, Nossent JC. Increased mortality in ankylosing spondylitis is related to disease activity. Ann Rheum Dis. 2011;70(11):1921-5.

47. Liew JW, Ramiro S, Gensler LS. Cardiovascular morbidity and mortality in ankylosing spondylitis and psoriatic arthritis. Best Pract Res Clin Rheumatol. 2018;32(3):369-89.

48. Prati C, Claudepierre P, Pham T, Wendling D. Mortality in spondylarthritis. Joint

Bone Spine. 2011;78(5):466-70.

49. Castaneda S, Nurmohamed MT, González Gay MA. Cardiovascular disease in inflammatory rheumatic diseases. Best Pract Res Clin Rheumatol. 2016;30(5):851-69.

50. Mathieu S, Soubrier M. Cardiovascular risk in spondyloarthritis axial. Presse Med. 2015;44(9):907-11.

51. Peters ML, Visman I, Nielen MJ, Van Dillen N, Verheij RA, Van Der Horst Bruinsma IE, et al. Ankylosing spondylitis: a risk factor for myocardial infarction: table 1. Ann Rheum Dis. 2010;69(3):579-81.

52. Eriksson JK, Jacobsson L, Bengtsson K, Askling J. Is ankylosing spondylitis a risk factor for cardiovascular disease, and how do these risks compare with those in rheumatoid arthritis? Ann Rheum Dis. 2017;76(2):364-70.

53. Huang YP, Wang YH, Pan SL. Increased risk of ischemic heart disease in young patients with newly diagnosed ankylosing spondylitis - a population-based longitudinal follow-up study. PLoS One. 2013;8(5):e64155.

54. Brophy S, Cooksey R, Atkinson M, Zhou SM, Husain MJ, Macey S, et al. No increased rate of acute myocardial infarction or stroke among patients with ankylosing spondylitis-a retrospective cohort study using routine data. Semin Arthritis Rheum. 2012;42(2):140-5.

55. Bosmans LA, Bosch L, Kusters PH, Lutgens E, Seijkens TP. The CD40-CD40L dyad as immunotherapeutic target in cardiovascular disease. J Cardiovasc Transl Res. 2021;14(1):13-22.

56. Arida A, Protogerou AD, Konstantonis G, Konsta M, Delicha EM, Kitas GD, et al. Subclinical atherosclerosis is not accelerated in patients with ankylosing spondylitis with low disease activity: new data and metaanalysis of published studies. J Rheumatol. 2015;42(11):2098-105.

57. Kucuk A, Ugur Uslu A, Icli A, Cure E, Arslan S, Turkmen K, et al. The LDL/HDL ratio and atherosclerosis in ankylosing spondylitis. Z Rheumatol. 2017;76(1):58-

63.

58. Choe JY, Lee MY, Rheem I, Rhee MY, Park SH, Kim SK. No differences of carotid intima-media thickness between young patients with ankylosing spondylitis and healthy controls. Joint Bone Spine. 2008;75(5):548-53.

59. Cure E, Icli A, Uslu AU, Sakiz D, Cure MC, Baykara RA, et al. Atherogenic index of plasma: a useful marker for subclinical atherosclerosis in ankylosing spondylitis: AIP associate with cIMT in AS. Clin Rheumatol. 2018;37(5):1273-80.

60. Ladehesa Pineda ML, Arias De La Rosa I, López Medina C, Castro Villegas MC, Ábalos Aguilera MC, Ortega Castro R, et al. Assessment of the relationship between estimated cardiovascular risk and structural damage in patients with axial spondyloarthritis. Ther Adv Musculoskelet Dis. 2020;12:1759720X20982837.

61. Rueda Gotor J, Quevedo Abeledo JC, Corrales A, Genre F, Hernández Hernández V, Delgado Frías E, et al. Reclassification into very-high cardiovascular risk after carotid ultrasound in patients with axial spondyloarthritis. Clin Exp Rheumatol. 2020;38(4):724-31.

62. Serdaroglu Beyazal M, Erdogan T, Türkyilmaz AK, Devrimsel G, Cüre MC, Beyazal M, et al. Relationship of serum osteoprotegerin with arterial stiffness, preclinical atherosclerosis, and disease activity in patients with ankylosing spondylitis. Clin Rheumatol. 2016;35(9):2235-41.

63. Resorlu H, Akbal A, Resorlu M, Gokmen F, Ates C, Uysal F, et al. Epicardial adipose tissue thickness in patients with ankylosing spondylitis. Clin Rheumatol. 2015;34(2):295-9.

64. Hamdi W, Chelli Bouaziz M, Zouch I, Ghannouchi MM, Haouel M, Ladeb MF, et al. Assessment of preclinical atherosclerosis in patients with ankylosing spondylitis. J Rheumatol. 2012;39(2):322-6.

65. Giollo A, Dalbeni A, Cioffi G, Ognibeni F, Gatti D, Idolazzi L, et al. Factors associated with accelerated subclinical atherosclerosis in patients with

spondyloarthritis without overt cardiovascular disease. Clin Rheumatol. 2017;36(11):2487-95.

66. Perrotta FM, Scarno A, Carboni A, Bernardo V, Montepaone M, Lubrano E, et al. Assessment of subclinical atherosclerosis in ankylosing spondylitis: correlations with disease activity indices. Reumatismo. 2013;65(3):105-12.

67. Singh T, Newman AB. Inflammatory markers in population studies of aging. Ageing Res Rev. 2011;10(3):319-29.

68. Gonzalez Juanatey C, Vazquez Rodriguez TR, Miranda Filloy JA, Dierssen T, Vaqueiro I, Blanco R, et al. The high prevalence of subclinical atherosclerosis in patients with ankylosing spondylitis without clinically evident cardiovascular disease. Medicine. 2009;88(6):358-65.

69. Sari I, Okan T, Akar S, Cece H, Altay C, Secil M, et al. Impaired endothelial function in patients with ankylosing spondylitis. Rheumatology. 2006;45(3):283-6.

70. Verma I, Syngle A, Krishan P, Garg N. Endothelial progenitor cells as a marker of endothelial dysfunction and atherosclerosis in ankylosing spondylitis: a cross-sectional study. Int J Angiol. 2016;26(01):036-42.

71. Bodnár N, Kerekes G, Seres I, Paragh G, Kappelmayer J, Némethné ZG, et al. Assessment of subclinical vascular disease associated with ankylosing spondylitis. J Rheumatol. 2011;38(4):723-9.

72. Erre GL, Mangoni AA, Castagna F, Paliogiannis P, Carru C, Passiu G, et al. Meta Analysis of asymmetric dimethylarginine concentrations in rheumatic diseases. Sci Rep. 2019;9:5426.

73. Berg IJ, Van Der Heijde D, Dagfinrud H, Seljeflot I, Olsen IC, Kvien TK, et al. Disease activity in ankylosing spondylitis and associations to markers of vascular pathology and traditional cardiovascular disease risk factors: a cross-sectional study. J Rheumatol. 2015;42(4):645-53.

74. Przepiera B⅛dzak H, Fischer K, Brzosko M. Serum interleukin-18, fetuin-a,

soluble intercellular adhesion molecule-1, and endothelin-1 in ankylosing spondylitis, psoriatic arthritis, and SAPHO syndrome. Int J Mol Sci. 2016;17(8):1255.

75. Wang HH, Wang QF. Low vaspin levels are related to endothelial dysfunction in patients with ankylosing spondylitis. Braz J Med Biol Res. 2016;49(7):e5231.

76. Resnick HE, Lindsay RS, McDermott MM, Devereux RB, Jones KL, Fabsitz RR, et al.

al. Relationship of high and low ankle brachial index to all-cause and cardiovascular disease mortality: the strong heart study. Circulation. 2004;109(6):733-9.

77. Zhu D, Mackenzie NW, Farquharson C, MacRae VE. Mechanisms and clinical consequences of vascular calcification. Front Endocrinol. 2012;3:95.

78. Del Rincon I, Haas RW, Pogosian S, Escalante A. Lower limb arterial incompressibility and obstruction in rheumatoid arthritis. Ann Rheum Dis. 2005;64(3):425-32.

79. Ding J, Ghali O, Lencel P, Broux O, Chauveau C, Devedjian JC, et al. TNF-α and IL-1β inhibits RUNX2 and collagen expression but increase alkaline phosphatase activity and mineralization in human mesenchymal stem cells. Life Sci. 2009;84(15):499-504.

80. Al Aly Z, Shao JS, Lai CF, Huang E, Cai J, Behrmann A, et al. Aortic msx2-wnt Calcification cascade is regulated by TNF-α-dependent signals in diabetic Ldlr / Mice. Arterioscler Thromb Vasc Biol. 2007;27(12):2589-96.

81. Tintut Y, Patel J, Parhami F, Demer LL. Tumor necrosis factor-α promotes in vitro calcification of vascular cells via the cAMP pathway. Circulation. 2000;102(21):2636-42.

82. Lencel P, Delplace S, Pilet P, Leterme D, Miellot F, Sourice S, et al. Cell-specific effects of TNF-α and IL-1β on alkaline phosphatase: implication for syndesmophyte formation and vascular calcification. Lab Invest.

2011;91(10):1434-42.

83. Guellec D, Bressollette L, Gueguen F, Jousse Joulin S, Marhadour T, Devauchelle Pensec V, et al. Is routine ankle-brachial pressure index evaluation useful in rheumatoid arthritis? Joint Bone Spine. 2013;80(1):111-3.

84. Bilim S, íçagasioglu A, Akbal A, Kasapoglu E, Gürsel S. Assessment of subclinical atherosclerosis with ankle-brachial index in psoriatic arthritis: a case-control study. Arch Rheumatol. 2021;36(2):210-8.

85. Agewall S. Is impaired flow-mediated dilatation of the brachial artery a cardiovascular risk factor? Curr Vasc Pharmacol. 2003;1(2):107-9.

86. Svanteson M, Rollefstad S, Kl0w NE, Hisdal J, Ikdahl E, Semb AG, et al. Associations between coronary and carotid artery atherosclerosis in patients with inflammatory joint diseases. RMD Open. 2017;3(2):e000544.

87. Celermajer DS, Sorensen KE, Spiegelhalter DJ, Georgakopoulos D, Robinson J, Deanfield JE. Aging is associated with endothelial dysfunction in healthy men years before the age-related decline in women. J Am Coll Cardiol. 1994;24(2):471-6.

88. Sasaki Y, Ikeda Y, Miyauchi T, Uchikado Y, Akasaki Y, Ohishi M. Estrogen-SIRT1 axis plays a pivotal role in protecting arteries against menopause-induced senescence and atherosclerosis. J Atheroscler Thromb. 2020;27(1):47-59.

89. Morovatdar N, Thrift AG, Stranges S, Kapral M, Behrouz R, Amiri A, et al. Socioeconomic status and long-term stroke mortality, recurrence and disability in iran: the mashhad stroke incidence study. Neuroepidemiology. 2019;53(1-2):27-31.

90. Manfredini R, De Giorgi A, Tiseo R, Boari B, Cappadona R, Salmi R, et al. Marital status, cardiovascular diseases, and cardiovascular risk factors: a review of the evidence. J Womens Health. 2017;26(6):624-32.

91. Celeng C, Takx RP, Lessmann N, Maurovich Horvat P, Leiner T, Isgum I, et al. The association between marital status, coronary computed tomography imaging biomarkers, and mortality in a lung cancer screening population. J

Thorac Imaging. 2020;35(3):204-9.

92. Konukoglu D, Uzun H. Endothelial dysfunction and hypertension. Adv Exp Med Biol. 2017;956:511-40.

93. Mathieu S, Joly H, Baron G, Tournadre A, Dubost JJ, Ristori JM, et al. Trend towards increased arterial stiffness or intima-media thickness in ankylosing spondylitis patients without clinically evident cardiovascular disease. Rheumatology. 2008;47(8):1203-7.

94. Malesci D, Niglio A, Mennillo GA, Buono R, Valentini G, La Montagna G. High prevalence of metabolic syndrome in patients with ankylosing spondylitis. Clin Rheumatol. 2007;26(5):710-4.

95. Hsu P, Lee W, Chiu C, Chen Y, Chang C, Tsai W, et al. Usefulness of ankle-brachial index calculated using diastolic blood pressure for prediction of mortality in patients with acute myocardial infarction. J Clin Hypertens. 2020;22(11):2044-50.

96. Skare TL, Verceze GC, Oliveira AA, Perreto S. Carotid intima-media thickness in spondyloarthritis patients. Sao Paulo Med J. 2013;131(2):100-5.

97. Kimhi O, Caspi D, Bornstein NM, Maharshak N, Gur A, Arbel Y, et al. Prevalence and risk factors of atherosclerosis in patients with psoriatic arthritis. Semin Arthritis Rheum. 2007;36(4):203-9.

98. Poddubnyy D, Haibel H, Listing J, Marker Hermann E, Zeidler H, Braun J, et al. Baseline radiographic damage, elevated acute-phase reactant levels, and cigarette smoking status predict spinal radiographic progression in early axial spondyloarthritis. Arthritis Rheum. 2012;64(5):1388-98.

99. Kang KY, Her YH, Ju JH, Hong YS, Park SH. Radiographic progression is associated with increased cardiovascular risk in patients with axial spondyloarthritis. Mod Rheumatol. 2016;26(4):601-6.

100. Vander Cruyssen B, Vastesaeger N, Collantes Estévez E. Hip disease in ankylosing spondylitis. Curr Opin Rheumatol. 2013;25(4):448-54.

101. Slimani S, Hamdi W, Nassar K, Kalla AA. Spondyloarthritis in north africa: an update. Clin Rheumatol. 2021;40(9):3401-10.

102. Patel ML, Sachan R, Singh GP, Chaudhary SC, Gupta KK, Atam V, et al. Assessment of subclinical atherosclerosis and endothelial dysfunction in chronic kidney disease by measurement of carotid intima media thickness and flow-mediated vasodilatation in north indian population. J Family Med Prim Care. 2019;8(4):1447-52.

103. Khandelwal P, Murugan V, Hari S, Lakshmy R, Sinha A, Hari P, et al. Dyslipidemia, carotid intima-media thickness and endothelial dysfunction in children with chronic kidney disease. Pediatr Nephrol. 2016;31(8):1313-20.

104. Schiffrin EL, Lipman ML, Mann JE. Chronic kidney disease: effects on the cardiovascular system. Circulation. 2007;116(1):85-97.

105. Hirakawa Y, Jao TM, Inagi R. Pathophysiology and therapeutics of premature ageing in chronic kidney disease, with a focus on glycative stress. Clin Exp Pharmacol Physiol. 2017;44(Suppl 1):70-7.

106. Abou Saleh H. Role of endothelial progenitor cells in the regulation of endothelial function.
of platelet function [Thesis]. Biomedical Sciences: Montreal; 2008. 188p.

107. Ruane O'Hora T, Markos F. Platelets do not alter flow-mediated dilation or arterial conduction in vivo. J Vasc Res. 2021;58(4):231-6.

108. Karabag T, Kaya A, Yavuz S, Kaya C, Koc F, Yeter E. The relation of HOMA index with endothelial functions determined by flow mediated dilatation method among hyperglycemic patients. Indian Heart J. 2007;59(6):463-7.

109. Acevedo M, Kramer V, Tagle R, Corbalán R, Arnaiz P, Berríos X, et al. Relación colesterol total a HDL y colesterol no HDL: los mejores indicadores lipidicos de aumento de grosor de la íntima media carotidea. Rev Med Chil. 2012;140(8):969-76.

110. Steinberg HO, Bayazeed B, Hook G, Johnson A, Cronin J, Baron AD. Endothelial

dysfunction is associated with cholesterol levels in the high normal range in humans. Circulation. 1997;96(10):3287-93.

111. Fichtlscherer S, Rosenberger G, Walter DH, Breuer S, Dimmeler S, Zeiher AM. Elevated C-reactive protein levels and impaired endothelial vasoreactivity in patients with coronary artery disease. Circulation. 2000;102(9):1000-6.

112. Kearney PM, Baigent C, Godwin J, Halls H, Emberson JR, Patrono C. Do selective cyclo-oxygenase-2 inhibitors and traditional non-steroidal antiinflammatory drugs increase the risk of atherothrombosis? Meta-analysis of randomised trials. Br Med J. 2006;332(7553):1302-8.

113. Braun J, Baraliakos X, Westhoff T. Nonsteroidal anti-inflammatory drugs and cardiovascular risk - a matter of indication. Semin Arthritis Rheum. 2020;50(2):285-8.

114. Végh E, Kerekes G, Pusztai A, Hamar A, Szamosi S, Váncsa A, et al. Effects of 1-year anti-TNF-α therapy on vascular function in rheumatoid arthritis and ankylosing spondylitis. Rheumatol Int. 2020;40(3):427-36.

115. Tam LS, Shang Q, Kun EW, Lee KL, Yip ML, Li M, et al. The effects of golimumab on subclinical atherosclerosis and arterial stiffness in ankylosing spondylitis--a randomized, placebo-controlled pilot trial. Rheumatology. 2014;53(6):1065-74.

116. Van Sijl AM, Van Eijk IC, Peters ML, Serné EH, Van Der Horst Bruinsma IE, Smulders YM, et al. Tumour necrosis factor blocking agents and progression of subclinical atherosclerosis in patients with ankylosing spondylitis. Ann Rheum Dis. 2015;74(1):119-23.

117. Angel K, Provan SA, Fagerhol MK, Mowinckel P, Kvien TK, Atar D. Effect of 1 year anti-TNF-α therapy on aortic stiffness, carotid atherosclerosis, and calprotectin in inflammatory arthropathies: a controlled study. Am J Hypertens. 2012;25(6):644-50.

118. Hokstad I, Deyab G, Wang Fagerland M, Lyberg T, Hjeltnes G, F0rre 0, et al. Tumor necrosis factor inhibitors are associated with reduced complement

activation in spondylarthropathies: an observational study. PLoS One. 2019;14(7):e0220079.

119. Capkin E, Karkucak M, Kiris A, Durmus I, Karaman K, Karaca A, et al. Anti-TNF-therapy may not improve arterial stiffness in patients with AS: a 24-week follow-up. Rheumatology. 2012;51(5):910-4.

120. Mathieu S, Pereira B, Couderc M, Rabois E, Dubost JJ, Soubrier M. No Significant changes in arterial stiffness in patients with ankylosing spondylitis after tumour necrosis factor alpha blockade treatment for 6 and 12 months. Rheumatology. 2013;52(1):204-9.

121. Szekanecz Z, Kerekes G, Soltész P. Vascular effects of biologic agents in RA and spondyloarthropathies. Nat Rev Rheumatol. 2009;5(12):677-84.

122. Gonzalez Juanatey C, Testa A, Garcia Castelo A, Garcia Porrua C, Llorca J, Gonzalez Gay MA. Active but transient improvement of endothelial function in rheumatoid arthritis patients undergoing long-term treatment with anti-tumor necrosis factor α antibody: anti-TNFα and endothelial function in RA. Arthritis Rheum. 2004;51(3):447-50.

123. Gonzalez Gay MA, Garcia Unzueta MT, De Matias JM, Gonzalez Juanatey C, Garcia Porrua C, Sanchez Andrade A, et al. Influence of anti-TNF-alpha infliximab therapy on adhesion molecules associated with atherogenesis in patients with rheumatoid arthritis. Clin Exp Rheumatol. 2006;24(4):373-9.

124. Knowles L, Nadeem N, Chowienczyk PJ. Do anti-tumour necrosis factor-α biologics affect subclinical measures of atherosclerosis and arteriosclerosis? A systematic review. Br J Clin Pharmacol. 2020;86(5):837-51.

125. Grosser T, Theken KN, Fitz Gerald GA. Cyclooxygenase inhibition: pain, inflammation, and the cardiovascular system. Clin Pharmacol Ther. 2017;102(4):611-22.

126. Schjerning AM, McGettigan P, Gislason G. Cardiovascular effects and safety of (non-aspirin) NSAIDs. Nat Rev Cardiol. 2020;17(9):574-84.

127. Agca R, Heslinga SC, Rollefstad S, Heslinga M, McInnes IB, Peters MJL, et al. EULAR recommendations for cardiovascular disease risk management in patients with rheumatoid arthritis and other forms of inflammatory joint disorders: 2015/2016 update. Ann Rheum Dis. 2017;76(1):17-28. DOI: 10.1136/annrheumdis-2016-209775

128. Lefferts EC, Hibner BA, Lefferts WK, Lima NS, Baynard T, Haus JM, et al. Oral vitamin C restores endothelial function during acute inflammation in young and older adults. Physiol Rep. 2021;9(21):e15104.

129. Changal KH, Khan MS, Bashir R, Sheikh MA. Curcumin preparations can improve flow-mediated dilation and endothelial function: a meta-analysis. Complement Med Res. 2020;27(4):272281.

130. Baigent C, Blackwell L, Emberson J, Holland LE, Reith C, Bhala N, et al. Efficacy and safety of more intensive lowering of LDL cholesterol: a meta-analysis of data from 170 000 participants in 26 randomised trials. Lancet. 2010;376(9753):1670-81.

131. Crouse JR, Raichlen JS, Riley WA, Evans GW, Palmer MK, O'Leary DH, et al. Effect of rosuvastatin on progression of carotid intima-media thickness in low-risk individuals with subclinical atherosclerosis: the meteor trial. J Am Med Assoc. 2007;297(12):1344.

132. Ridker PM, Wilson PF, Grundy SM. Should C-reactive protein be added to metabolic syndrome and to assessment of global cardiovascular risk? Circulation. 2004;109(23):2818-25.

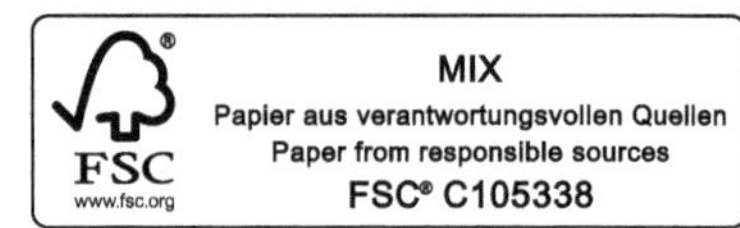

Printed by Books on Demand GmbH, Norderstedt / Germany